Royal Earlswood

A history

Anne Lea

Vice-Chair

On behalf of the Royal Earlswood Museum Committee.

Published by Anne Lea

©   Anne Lea

ISBN   0-9550613-0-X

Printed by Netherne Printers

2005

Front cover: Front view of Royal Earlswood

CONTENTS

Author's Note

Terminology used to describe people with a Learning Disability has changed several times since Earlswood first opened in 1855. Although terms such as 'idiot and 'imbecile' are no longer in favour it should be remembered that they were, and remain, medical descriptions of degrees of handicap, being based on the assessments of a person's Intelligence Quotient (I.Q.). When planning this volume it was decided to use, as far as possible, the terminology in common usage during the period under discussion.

The information contained within this volume has generally been collected from secondary and even tertiary sources. As such there will be errors, despite efforts to confirm details where possible. The author apologises in advance for any such errors and would be pleased to hear from anyone in a position to provide corrections.

Acknowledgements

The author would like to thank the Freda Knight, Chair, Sylvia McFarlane, Secretary, and all the members of the Royal Earlswood Museum Committee for all their help and support during the writing of this history. Thanks go especially to my husband for his help and patience, and especially for his computer wizardry!

FOREWORD

I have great pleasure in introducing this definitive history of the Royal Earlswood, pioneering hospital and home for people with learning disabilities, which started as a project for the Royal Earlswood Museum Committee. Anne Lea bravely took on this onerous commitment and has done a marvellous job.

The Royal Earlswood Museum was started in the 1960s by senior psychologist Diana Cortazzi, when she began collecting items of historical interest scattered around the building. Much of the archive had been lost or neglected, and she realised how important it was to salvage what remained. With the help of staff volunteers, she created a small museum, and eventually the management secured a grant from the King Edward's Hospital Fund towards a purpose built museum, attached to the social club in the grounds. It was opened in 1967, and its aim was to provide material to aid study, research and education, but to be entertaining as well as instructive. It was opened and shown to staff and visitors on request by volunteers, but over the years it became rather neglected.

When the date for closure of Royal Earlswood was confirmed, the Chief Executive, Martin Barkley asked that interested staff form a committee to try to find a way forward for the museum. Over the next two years the Chairman of the Trust and museum committee tried to find alternative accommodation, without success. Then, a few weeks before closure, committee secretary Sylvia McFarlane alerted Mary Waller, then Mayor of Reigate and Banstead, to the plight of the museum. At the eleventh hour, she brokered an arrangement for accommodation in the Belfry Shopping Centre, Redhill, with manager, Paul Alcock, and with the permission of the freeholders, the Prudential. Two display areas were made available on Car Park Level One, which enabled some of the most interesting and attractive artefacts to be exhibited behind glass. Thanks to these people, an important part of Redhill's history was saved.

In June 1997, this previously "hidden museum" was opened to the public, and like the residents, came out into the community. Although only 10% of the museum artefacts are on display, the remainder being in store, hundreds of people are now able to enjoy this unusual exhibition when they are shopping in the Belfry –

probably the first museum in a shopping centre.

Freda Knight
Chairman, Royal Earlswood Museum Committee

May 2005.

The Foundation of an Institution.

When the doors of Royal Earlswood finally closed on the 31st of March 1997 it marked the end of an organisation with a history going back one hundred and fifty years.

Earlswood was the first hospital of its kind in Britain. It owed its existence to the foresight, understanding and concern of one woman and a small group of philanthropists. Mrs. Anne Serina Plumbe lived in Whitechapel, London and was the mother of a disabled son. She was dismayed by the plight of the feeble-minded children in the area. Early in 1847 her husband Samuel read an article in the *'Chambers Journal'*, written by Mr. Gaskell of Lancaster County Lunatic Asylum. It described the work of Dr. Itard, Dr. Voisin and the Bicêtre Hospital in Paris where such children had been accommodated and educated since 1828. Mrs. Plumbe contacted Gaskell for further information and then wrote over 600 letters to people who she hoped would be interested. Mrs. Plumbe applied to Dr. Reed, her local clergyman, for assistance.

Dr. Andrew was born in 1787 and had been initially trained to follow in his father's profession. However, he found that his own inclination lay in the direction of the church and he was finally ordained in 1811. He was concerned for the welfare of the poor and by 1847 had already founded three orphanages. From 1837 onwards there are mentions in his private writings of the need for an Idiot Asylum. Samuel Plumbe was one of his earliest and best friends and colleagues. He had been born in Tiverton, Devon. On moving to London he took a prominent place in Dr. Reed's church, Wycliffe Chapel in Commercial Road.

Dr. Reed wished to confirm the need for an institution. He agreed to pursue the matter if Mrs. Plumbe could locate six 'idiot' children within six days. She found 28 boys, most in a wretched state. True to his promise Andrew Reed turned his attention to the plight of these children. At that time, generally the only recourse for a family with such a child was to place them in the workhouse or a lunatic asylum, or have them 'boarded out' in private homes. Care could be indifferent, at best. Little attention was paid to the improvement of the individuals' condition.

The difference between mental defect and mental disease was recognised at the time of Edward I, though it was crudely defined. The one being a "born fool" whilst the other was a person who "hath had understanding, but by disease, grief or other accident has lost the use of his reason."

In 1815 'idiocy' was first distinguished from 'lunacy' for the purposes of treatment. However, it was not until 1886 that local authorities were permitted to provide special asylums, and few did so. It is, therefore, all the more remarkable that a small group of men, led by Dr. Reed, met on the twentieth of July 1847, in the 'King's Head Tavern', Poultry, London, to discuss the need for a separate and distinct institution for the benefit of the 'idiot'. It was agreed to publish the proposal for the institution in certain leading journals. At the meeting Dr. Reed said that:

> **"...the care of the Idiot ought to be perfectly distinct from that of the insane, and that much might be done for his education; and he was anxious to ascertain by free conference with benevolent persons, whether an attempt might not be made to establish an Institution for their separate and especial benefit."**

Mrs. Plumbe meanwhile began a correspondence with Dr. John Conolly on the topic of an asylum. He was a progressive psychiatrist and Resident Physician of Hanwell Lunatic Asylum in Middlesex. He was already famous for his work with the insane. Unlike many of his fellow doctors he was a firm believer that much could be achieved without the need for mechanical restraints. He shared with Dr. Reed the philosophy that, with careful teaching, the majority of 'idiots' were capable of improvement.

Institutions already existed in France, Switzerland, Germany, Scandinavia and America. In 1846 a school had been set up in Belvedere Street, Bath by two sisters, 'the Misses White'. However, they took only a small number of paying patients. Dr. Reed corresponded with medical men in a number of countries and travelled across Europe to gather information. He also set about investigating the actual condition of the idiot in the workhouses and lunatic asylums of England and Wales. A survey of lunatic asylums conducted around 1857 indicates what he must have found. Of 33,000 inmates, 14,000 were mentally ill whilst the majority were 'idiots'. At best they were detained for their own protection, at worst for the comfort of society. Measures to combat their disability or improve their skills were impracticable.

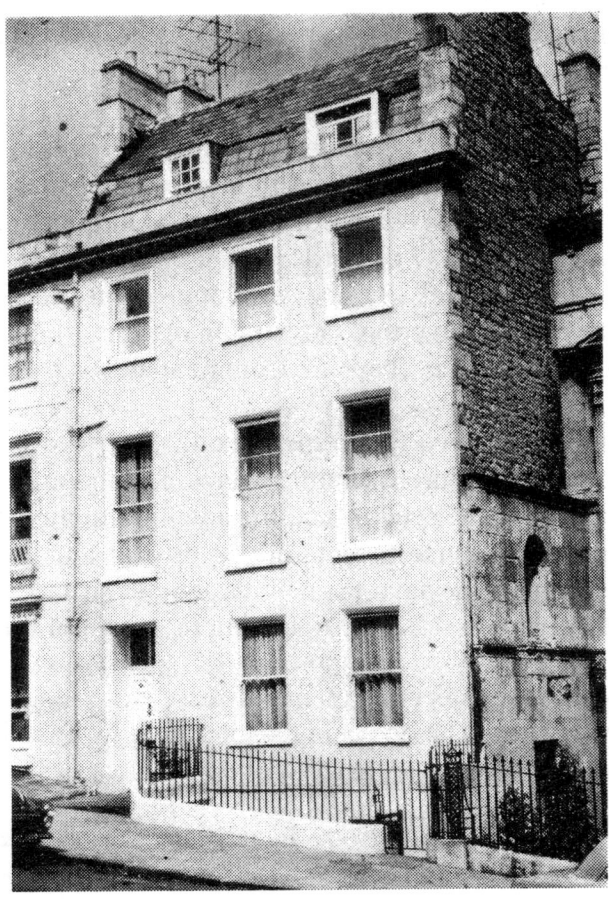

The 'Misses White' House in Bath

By September 1847 Lord Palmerston had been persuaded to join the project. At a Public Meeting held on the twenty-seventh of October 1847 at the 'London Tavern' in Bishopsgate Street, the Charity was established as 'The National Association for Asylum for Idiots'. The officers were to include Lord Palmerston, the Right Honourable Lord Ashley, Sir George Carroll, Lord Mayor of London, Baron Rothschild, Dr. Reed and Dr. Conolly. Also on the first Asylum Board was Sir James Clarke, physician to Queen Victoria. The funds were to be raised by subscription and the Rules and Constitution of the new society were read. The text of the address was:

"We plead for those who cannot plead for themselves."

The constitution was laid down with the aim:

> **"not merely to take the Idiot under its care, but especially, by the skilful and earnest application of the best means in his education, to prepare, as far as possible, *for the duties and enjoyments of life,* the Idiot, who,......was likely to derive benefit from the treatment without restriction as to age, sex or country."**

By November 1847 the Charity had rented offices at 29, Poultry for the sum of £60 per annum. From the 22nd of November the Board met at this address and began the search for a suitable house for the Asylum.

Postscript: Mrs. Plumbe's son, Andrew Reed Plumbe, was admitted to the new Asylum in 1848. He died of tuberculosis in Earlswood on the 20th of March 1881, aged 45. Mrs. Plumbe continued to be a supporter of the Charity. She died in 1883 at the age of 83 years and left a legacy of 19 guineas to Earlswood.

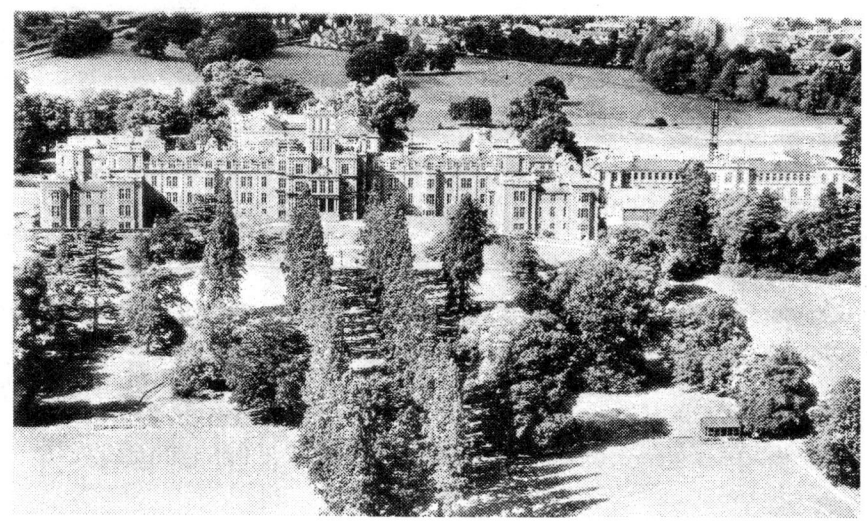

Earlswood from the air.

Park House.

Having decided to proceed with the Asylum, the Committee required a building in which to house their charges. Several properties were considered and negotiations for one were attempted unsuccessfully. The Committee finally settled on a Regency manor in Highgate called Park House. In March 1848 a lease was purchased for 11 years at £250 per annum. Even before the documents were signed, arrangements had been made to have the house decorated. By the end of March some furniture had been purchased at a sale on the premises at Highgate.

The estate belonged to a Mr. Cooper and had been the site of the Highgate Brewery since about 1670. W.D.C.Cooper was an influential man in Highgate and took an interest in the community. He was chairman of the governors of Highgate School, on the management committee of the local National School and welcomed the meetings of the Book Society at his house. He was a magistrate in Middlesex and in Bedfordshire, where he was also Deputy Lieutenant. He was a philanthropist. He provided allotments on his land in Toddington to alleviate the suffering of rural labourers who had lost their land as a result of the Enclosure Acts. On his death in 1860 these amounted to 3,388 acres.

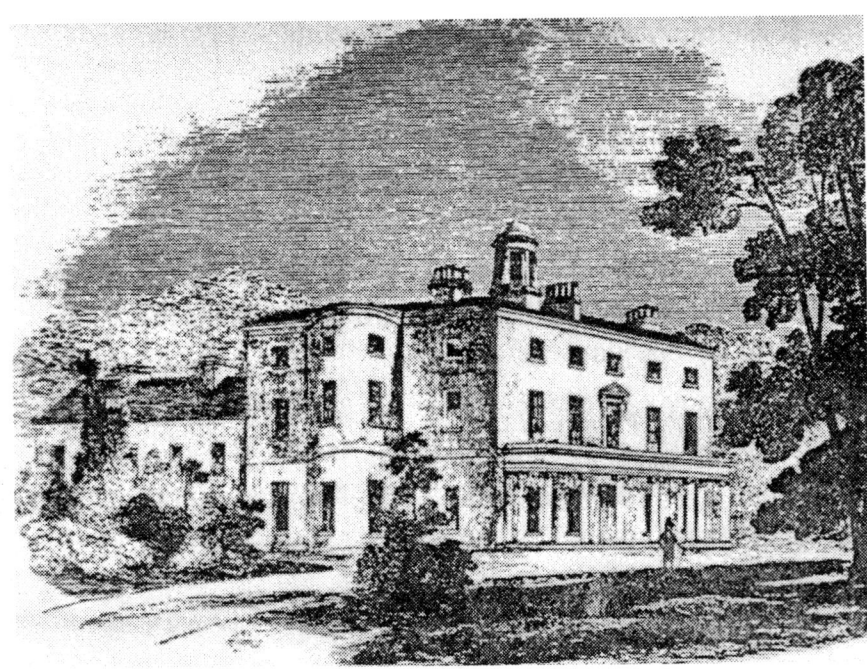

Park House
(Reprinted courtesy of Camden Local Studies and Archives Centre)

Park House was a substantial mansion. It was sited on the crown of Highgate Hill in the middle of sixteen acres of pleasure grounds and gardens. The main entrance faced North Hill and was screened from it by huge elm trees. The building was almost square except for a large bay on the north side. On the west side a portico with six pillars extended across the full width of the house. The east wing had a conservatory built along the south side. It had three storeys topped off by a domed turret. A similar sized building to the northeast housed a coach house and stables. During the time that the Asylum occupied the estate, a single storey building was constructed to link the two structures. This was probably used as a laundry.

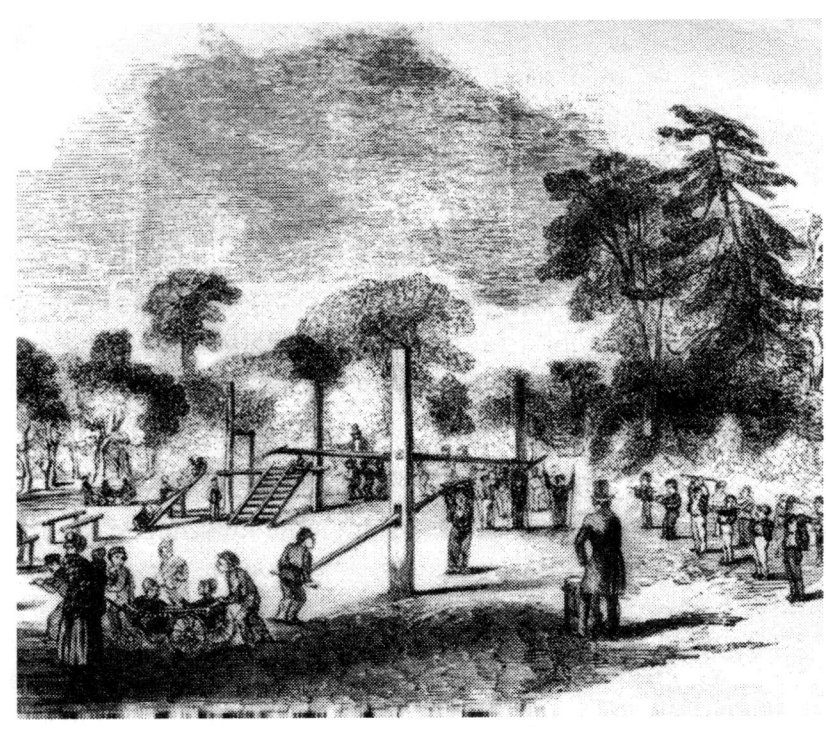

Park House playground
(Reprinted courtesy of Camden Local Studies and Archives Centre)

4

In April 1848 the first staff were engaged. Mr. Millard was appointed as Superintendent and schoolmaster of the Asylum at an annual salary of £100 plus board and lodgings. He was a friend of Mrs. Plumbe and had been Honorary Superintendent of a 'ragged school'. Miss Cockburn was appointed as matron at £40 per year. In May Mr. Harrington joined the staff as singing and gymnastics master. He received £60 per annum in return for three four-hour sessions per week. By December this had been increased to five days from 9am to 4.30pm and the salary to £100 per annum.

The first 17 patients arrived on the 26th of April 1848, a further child a few days later. Several rooms downstairs had been adapted to form a schoolroom. Here the children were to receive instruction in drawing and singing. Upstairs the floors had been converted into dormitories. A large play area was laid out at the rear of the house, equipped with swings and other activities.

In June 1848 Mr. Lynne was engaged as assistant teacher. His salary of £40 while boarding in the house rose to £70 when he boarded out. He resigned after only five months. Other staff employed included:

One cook	£15 per annum.
1 kitchen maid	£ 9 per annum.
1 housemaid	£10 per annum.
1 head attendant	£25 per annum.
2 attendants	£20 per annum each.
1 head nurse	£20 per annum.
2 nurses	£10 per annum each.

The staff, at this time, had responsibility for 33 residents, 30 males and 3 females.

A House Committee met for the first time on the 28th of June 1848. It addressed such practical matters as the supply of water and gas, and the provision of clothes for the residents. Also considered were the visiting arrangements for friends and relatives, as well as inspection of the Asylum by visitors. Plans were made to convert the stable block and coach house into a washing room, workshop, playroom and infirmary. Tenders were to be taken for supplies and it was agreed that gas lighting should be installed in the house.

The first Resident Medical Superintendent, Dr. Foreman, was appointed in October 1848. The salary of £200 per annum was to increase as the Asylum grew. Dr. Foreman was also provided with suitable accommodation for himself and one servant but was to find his own provisions.

Suitable staff was not always easy to find. Four attendants were dismissed in the second half of 1848, one for striking several children and another because of his violent temper and harsh treatment of his charges. The salary paid to the attendants was increased in December 1848 to £25. By March 1849 there were 53 residents and five attendants were employed. In autumn 1849 Miss Allow was engaged as teacher in the girls' school at £20 per annum. For this sum she had responsibility for the care of 18 children, as the young boys were included in the girls' school.

In March 1849 Prince Albert visited the site to inspect the progress of the charity and was favourably impressed. A year after the opening of Park House Andrew Reed wrote:

"There is now order, obedience to authority, classification, improvement and cheerful occupation. Windows are safe, boundaries are observed without walls

and doors are safe without locks. The desire now is not to get away but to stay. They are essentially not only an improving but a happy family. And all this is secured without the aid of correction or coercion."

The success of such a progressive institution threatened to be its downfall as the demand for places soared. The home was originally established for about forty residents. In May 1849 the Committee was so concerned about overcrowding that they began to look for a second house locally. However, a clause in the Act of Parliament relating to asylums stated, "an additional building must not be separated from the licensed house by intervening grounds".

By July 1849 the number of inmates had risen to 66, 54 boys and twelve girls. The opening of a second institution at Essex Hall was only a temporary respite. By 1851 the number had increased to 71, 58 males between the ages of five and 27 years and thirteen females aged six to 26. In addition the Institution continued to have problems attracting sufficient nurses of the desired quality. Andrew Reed decided that the only solution was a purpose built asylum. A site just outside Redhill was chosen.

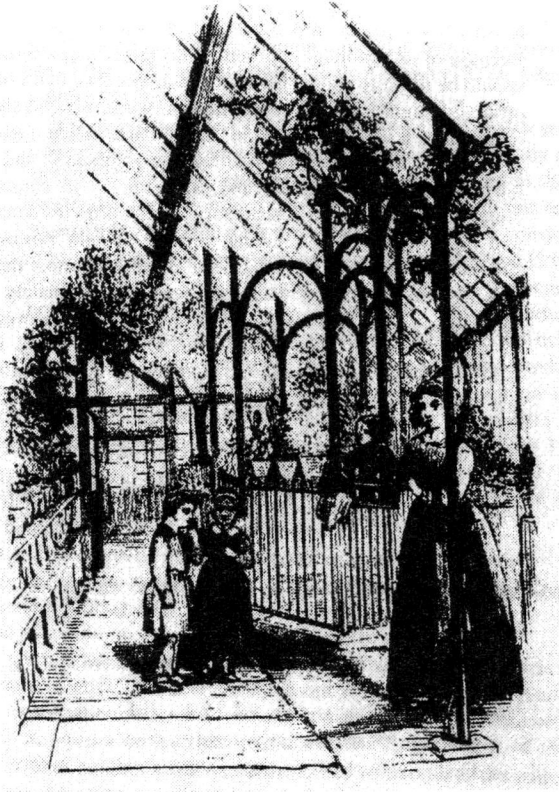

Park House, the covered walkway
(Reprinted courtesy of Camden Local Studies and Archives Centre)

There is no doubt that the establishment of the Charity had an impact on the treatment of 'idiots' in general. Dr. Hitchman, Medical Officer for Hanwell Lunatic Asylum, visited Park House in 1849 and shortly afterwards appointed a Master and Mistress "especially for the education of the idiotic portion of our large family."

In September 1855 Park House was closed and the furniture transferred to Earlswood. Andrew Reed felt some sadness at this move and wrote:

"September 1855. – Took farewell of Highgate. Regretted the place as the cradle of the idiot, the beautiful garden as improved under our care, and the fine old chestnut, our roof-tree, in all its glory."

In late 1855 the Church Penitentiary Association acquired the lease. For the following 80 years the Highgate 'House of Mercy' rescued prostitutes from a life of vice and misery. It helped them to reform and become useful members of the community. The residents were mainly teenagers and the life they had led was beyond the experience of most Victorian women. This fascinated and attracted many wealthy visitors to Park House. One of the regular visitors was the poet Christina Rossetti. She stayed at Park House for several weeks each year and insights gained there may have inspired some of her works. She threw herself into the experience totally, dressing in the nun-like black habit of a sister, with hanging sleeves, a muslin cap with lace edging and a veil. She was even offered the post of Lady Superintendent, which she declined. Her sister Maria also stayed there at least once and was later to become a nun.

Essex Hall.

Samuel Morton Peto, MP, a Vice President of the charity, initially solved the problem of overcrowding at Highgate. He resided at Somerleyton Hall in the County of Suffolk. Since the birth of the project he had been determined to do something for the 'idiots' of the Eastern Counties, but he was concerned that this should not be seen as rivalry. However, by 1850 the Charity had a waiting list of 170. He realised that the problems at Park House were becoming serious and made available a house near Colchester that he had purchased for between £1,200 and £1,400.

Essex Hall was in the Parish of Lexden, in the Borough of Colchester, and had originally been a hotel. Andrew Reed wrote on January 1st 1850:

> **"Very busy taking possession of Essex Hall, and moving a division of the family down. The work has increased at Highgate; it has now commenced at Colchester."**

The formal lease for Essex Hall was drawn up between Samuel Peto and nine representatives of the Charity. These included Andrew Reed, Dr. John Conolly and Dr. William Little. The lease was to run from Christmas Day 1849 for a period of seven, fourteen or twenty-one years at the option of the lessees. The rent was agreed at £320 per annum. However, for the same period Mr. Peto undertook to contribute £200 per annum to the Charity. In addition he advanced £1,000 towards the cost of fitting out the new home. This was to be repaid in seven years, without interest. On the 23rd of April 1852 Samuel Peto cancelled the loan and granted the money to the Charity as a gift.

The Board appointed staff for the new venture. It was decided that only the younger elected pupils should be transferred to Essex Hall. The family and friends of those to be transferred were consulted and all agreed to the change. Nineteen children travelled to Colchester with a schoolmaster, an assistant master and some attendants on Tuesday 8th of January 1850.

The Committee was eager to obtain further land in the vicinity of Essex Hall. Samuel Peto again came to their aid. He purchased a strip of land, adjoining the institution, from the Eastern Counties Railway Company. In a lease dated the 1st of March 1850 he agreed to transfer this to the Charity for the same term as the main property. The annual rent was to be 'a peppercorn'. In return the Asylum was to fence the said land within six months and maintain it.

Things did not go smoothly in the early days at Colchester. On the 3rd of May 1850 Andrew Reed wrote:

"Few infant charities have had so much to contend with- In two years, we have been burnt out, blown down, and robbed: besides which, our whole course was on untrodden ground. We had not been at Colchester a month when the terrible storm of the 7th of February occurred. It shattered the windows and doors, blew down two stacks of chimneys, crushing in roofs and floors. The poor people were up all night, and were safe from harm. What evil we were spared! I arrived in the morning to find the place a ruin. We first thanked God the Preserver; and then, the country-side was scoured for plumbers, glaziers, carpenters and builders."

In April 1851 the Reverend Edward Sidney of Cornard Parva visited Essex Hall. He reported in the press that:

"It is a happy discovery that the neglected idiot has a mind capable of improvement in its degree, and of a knowledge of a hope beyond this world.... Of all the wondrous projects of the present age, there is not one more worthy of Christian love, or with more encouraging prospects of success. I saw more than enough fully to convince me that it is worthy of the most cordial support."

Reverend Sidney described the children, sitting on benches in the schoolroom, attended by a "patient and gentle schoolmaster". Though most appeared unaware of their surroundings they came alive for the singing lesson. He questioned four of the most promising about the New Testament. Whilst he did not find any depth of understanding, he was stuck by the degree to which "this improvement of their limited faculties is attended with an unquestionable increase in happiness."

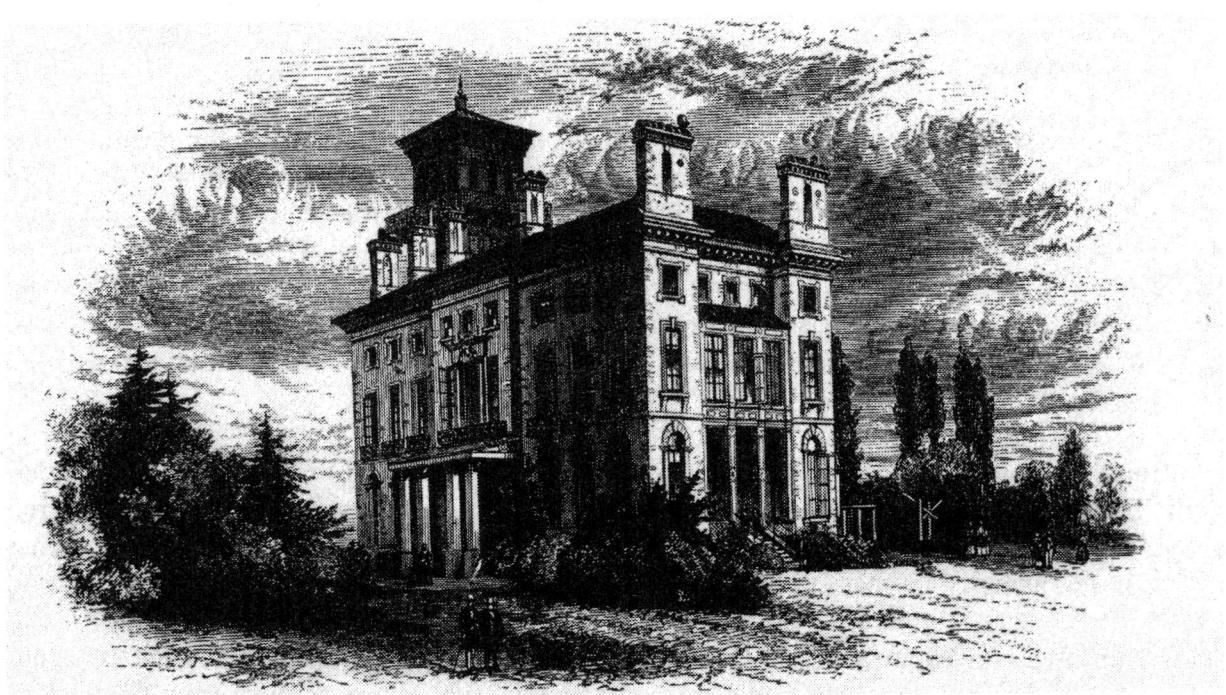

Essex Hall – The Idiot Asylum at Colchester

He witnessed the teaching of numbers and simple arithmetic. He saw the pleasure that was taken in drawing and the proficiency of seven or eight boys as they marched and went through their drill. Swings, ladders and gymnastic exercises were practised to the great benefit of health, mobility and mental state. He was especially impressed with the way that the older pupils were being taught a trade,

> **"One boy, who could not speak plainly, could not tell where he came from, and all his replies to questions manifested what he was, had, nevertheless, just put a large pane into one of the windows as perfectly as a regular glazier."**

Many of the residents of Essex Hall originated from the local area. Andrew Reed hoped that the Eastern Counties would accept responsibility for Essex Hall when the new Asylum in Redhill was ready for occupation. On the 23rd of May 1854 a meeting was convened with some of the more influential residents of the Eastern Counties. Plans were made to separate Essex Hall from its parent institution at Earlswood. It was to be managed and supported by the counties of Essex, Norfolk, Suffolk and Cambridge. All those residents who did not come from these four counties were to be transferred to Earlswood in the summer of 1855. Unfortunately, the committee that had been set up for the furtherance of this scheme ultimately refused to take over the institution. Essex Hall became a branch asylum of the main institution in Surrey.

Although unable to proceed immediately with his plan Andrew Reed continued to hope that the Eastern Counties would eventually agree to take responsibility for Essex Hall. Subscriptions of £1,000 per annum derived from the neighbourhood of Colchester. Dr. Reed was aware that much of this might be lost when the object of local interest was removed. Counties had undertaken to provide for the needs of their 'lunatic' population and Dr. Reed pleaded that the claims of the idiot were no less just. However, in October 1858 it was finally decided to close the home at Colchester. All seventy-five patients were transferred to Earlswood, together with their furniture and belongings.

Essex Hall was finally instituted as a separate organisation, the Eastern Counties Idiot Asylum, on the 1st of February 1859. On the 18th of that month Andrew Reed wrote:

> **"Happy day! Essex Hall is saved, and the Eastern Counties Idiot Asylum is established."**

The Essex Telegraph of the 8th of March 1864 recorded the final purchase of the building although £150 was still to be found. The pattern of subscriptions and elections followed the model of its founding institution. However, the elections were to be held in January and July to separate them from those of Earlswood. By March 1864 the Eastern Counties Idiot Asylum had 97 inmates.

The Founder.

> **"We plead for those who cannot plead for themselves"**
>
> **"To elevate the idiot from existence to life – from animal being to manhood – from vacancy and unconsciousness to reason and reflection – to disimprison his soul that he might qualify to know his maker and look beyond our present imperfect modes of being to perfect life in a glorious and everlasting future"**
> *Andrew Reed D.D.*

When Andrew Reed founded the Asylum for Idiots, it was the fourth of five important charitable foundations for which he was responsible. The son of a watchmaker, he was originally trained to follow in his father's footsteps. However, he quickly realised that his route through life was to be very different.

Andrew Reed was descended from an old Norfolk family. Several of his ancestors had held office as Mayor of Norwich. His father, also called Andrew, was born in Dorset. The family were pious non-conformists. Accompanied by his father and brothers, Andrew senior walked sixteen miles every Sunday to attend early service at Bridport. He was the only one of six brothers to be trained in a mechanical trade. He moved from his birthplace to set up as a watchmaker in London. There he met his future wife Mary Ann Mullen. Following the death of her parents, Mary Ann had opened a small Dame School and gave much of her spare time to acts of charity. Once married they occupied part of Beaumont House in Butcher Row, St. Clement Dane's, near Temple Bar. Andrew carried on his trade in a large attic whilst his wife received her pupils in the drawing room below.

Born on the 27th of November 1787, Andrew was their fourth child but the first to survive beyond infancy. He later gained a sister Martha. Andrew's parents believed in the importance of education. Although it required a great sacrifice on their part they found a good school for Andrew in Colebrook Row, Islington. Inseparable from her brother, a school was found for Martha in the same neighbourhood.

At fifteen Andrew left home and became officially apprenticed to a watchmaker. However, his new life led him into temptations. In 1803 he recorded in his diary that he had twice attended the playhouse. At sixteen he turned his back on the 'bad company' he felt he had fallen into. His indentures cancelled, he returned home to resume work with his father.

Andrew senior was involved with the establishment of a Congregational movement and his son became a member of the church on his sixteenth birthday. Mary had a great desire to see Andrew ordained and in 1807 arranged for him to enter Hackney College. On his twenty-fourth birthday Andrew was ordained and became Minister of the New Road Chapel in London. In 1816 Andrew married Elizabeth, the elder daughter of Jasper Thomas Holmes of Castle Hill, Reading.

It was as a result of his work that he became aware of the inadequate provision made for orphans. In 1813, only two years after his ordination, he launched his first appeal. He gathered together a group of friends and the 'East London Orphan Asylum and Working School' was founded. In 1815 the name was changed to the 'London Orphan Asylum'. Over the next few years Andrew was successful in gaining Royal Patronage for his charity.

Once the London Orphan Asylum was well established Andrew's attention turned to another project he had been considering for some time. The founding of the 'Infant Orphan Asylum' took place in 1827. This grew slowly at first but in June 1841 the Prince Consort laid the foundation stone for a new, larger Asylum at Wanstead. This began an association between the two men that was to last for the rest of Prince Albert's life. Only two years later, a disagreement over the religious services practised at 'The Royal Wanstead School', as it was now known, led to Dr. Reed's resignation from the Board. In 1844 Andrew founded a new school for orphans in Richmond, 'The Asylum for Fatherless Children'. Moving first to Hackney, the school then transferred to an old mansion in Stamford Hill. Ultimately, an estate at Coulsdon, Surrey was acquired in 1853 and a new building was erected for the school, now known as 'Reedham'.

The mallet used for the laying of the foundation stone at Wanstead was carved from a piece of oak from the old Elizabethan Royal Exchange. An inscription was engraved on a silver plaque and the mallet was presented to the Prince as a memento. It was to gain four more plaques when it was used by the Prince Consort, and subsequently the Prince of Wales, to lay the foundation stones for Reedham School, the new building for the London Orphan Asylum, The Hospital for Incurables and also …Earlswood. The mallet was eventually presented to Andrew Reed's earliest foundation, by this time known as 'Reed's School', by Major Norman Brett-James. The school contacted all the other charities and offered the loan of the mallet for the laying of any future foundation stones.

> **"This mallet, made of**
> **The Oak**
> **of the former Royal Exchange,**
> **was used by**
> **H.R.H. PRINCE ALBERT**
> **in the laying of the first stone of the**
> **INFANT ORPHAN ASYLUM**
> **at Wanstead,**
> **June 2nd. 1841."**
>
> **"EARLSWOOD,**
> **H.R.H. THE PRINCE ALBERT,**
> **16th. June 1852."**
>
> **"REEDHAM,**
> **5th. August, 1856."**
>
> **"LONDON ORPHAN ASYLUM,**
> **H.R.H. THE PRINCE OF WALES,**
> **15TH. July, 1869."**
>
> **"HOSPITAL FOR INCURABLES,**
> **H.R.H. THE PRINCE OF WALES,**
> **7th. July 1879."**

Inscription on the Mallet

Andrew's interest in those with Mental Deficiency began as early as 1837 and culminated with the founding of the Asylum for Idiots in 1847. During this work Andrew Reed became aware of the plight of those who "by Disease, Accident or Deformity are hopelessly disqualified from the Duties of Life." In 1854 he began to consider the foundation of an institution for their care. His final foundation was initially based in Carshalton and then moved to a building in the grounds of Reedham. It was ultimately to become known as the 'Royal Hospital and Home for Incurables' at Putney.

Dr. Reed's interest did not end with the foundation of the charities. He continued his close involvement with the last three foundations, working tirelessly to educate the public. He encouraged men of substance to contribute financially to the organisations. He utilised the press to stimulate public interest and support nationally. Dr. Reed was also actively involved in the management of the establishments. Before the opening of Park House he spent many weeks preparing for the reception of the first inmates. He remembered the chaos of those early days:

> **"It was a spectacle unique in itself, sufficiently discouraging to the most**
> **resolved, and not to be forgotten in the after-time by any. It was a period of**

distraction, disorder and noise of the most unnatural character. Some had defective sight; most had no power of articulation; many were lame in limb or in muscle; and all were of weak and perverted mind. Some had been spoiled, some neglected, some ill-used. Some were clamorous without speech, and rebellious without mind; some were sullen and perverse, and some unconscious and inert. Some were constantly making involuntary noises from nervous irritation, and others hid themselves in corners from the face of man as from the face of the enemy. Windows were smashed, wainscoting broken, boundaries defied, and the spirit of lawlessness was triumphant. It seemed to me as though nothing less than the accommodations of a prison would meet the wants of such a family. Some who witnessed the scene retired from it in disgust, and others in despair; but from the very outset my young friend Millard(i) was a faithful coadjutor."

Although money was never plentiful it was spent well on providing the best for the residents. Andrew Reed involved himself in the selection of master, nurses and servants. He checked all contracts for supplies. He supervised the fitting of baths of all sorts, shower, douche and aromatic, the preparation of a gymnasium and provision of garden allotments. He spent many hours observing and recording the improvements that occurred and the treatments that were most efficacious.

Eventually, with gentle methods, good care and perseverance, the residents gradually responded and their health and mental state improved. Dr. Reed was convinced of the benefit of the care offered by the staff.

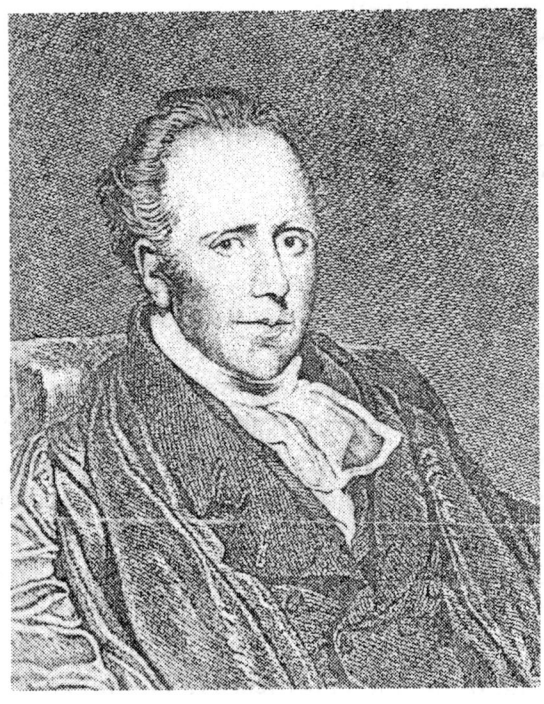

Andrew Reed D.D.

"I am convinced that, with such tending, one out of every three of the children may be greatly restored: and, if my good-will may avail, they shall be the merriest family in green England"

The smallest thing could produce a marvellous response in the children. One day Dr. Reed came across a child sobbing over a dead bird in the garden. He had never before been known to

(i) Superintendent at Park House

exhibit any emotion but the death of his favourite robin left him inconsolable. When Andrew Reed returned home he described the situation to his grandchildren who immediately offered their own pigeon house. The following day this was transported to Park House and Dr. Reed was there to introduce the birds to their enthusiastic, new friends. Over the years numerous animals found their way into the Asylum and helped to bring the experience of love to many.

> **"Never has anything within my observation grown so rapidly; never have I participated in graver responsibilities; never was the public more disposed to sympathise in the benevolent object. It satisfies my heart; the one link of charity that was wanting seems to be supplied at last; we have reached down to the lowest and most abandoned of the human family. Whatever comes of the effort this good will follow, England never again can neglect, scorn or incarcerate the poor idiot."**

> *Andrew Reed D.D.*

When Essex Hall opened Andrew Reed was principally responsible for the day-to-day management. Few others could spare the time to attend regularly an Asylum so far from London. He came so frequently that the children knew his name better than their own. He shared their meals, joined their games and never failed to visit those who were unable to leave their rooms.

Dr. Reed was already 60 years old when the charity was first founded. Such efforts took their toll on his health. In 1851 this was brought home to him.

> **"I had a strong intimation of my frailty and dependence. As I was going to Coulsdon, [Reedham School] I had an attack on my left side. I found suddenly that I could not button my coat; my arm and hand became disobedient, and a general numbness crept about me. I made my way to the Asylum; stood straight up, and resolved to be well; did my work; went to the Idiot Office in the Poultry for two hours; put things in train for a fortnight; and then hurried home to seek advice and medicine.... Submissively I pleaded that, just now, I would not faint and die. Just now, the two Asylums seem to have a special claim upon me."**

Andrew Reed was sent abroad to convalesce. However, he found himself unable to forget his charges. He toured Europe studying the advances being made in the treatment of the 'idiot'. He visited Germany, Denmark and Sweden. He was received by the King of Sweden and met with Professors of Medical Science and Natural Philosophy. On returning home he found a letter waiting for him from America, from a gentleman who had visited Park House and reported the establishment of an Asylum on the British model.

Returning to his labours Dr. Reed spent even Christmas Day at Essex Hall. He observed the delight with which the residents viewed the tree and enjoyed their meal of roast beef and plum pudding. He was impressed by the way the food was spread before the inmates and yet none made any effort to take it until grace had been sung.

When the Asylum at Earlswood was being built Dr. Reed purchased Earlsmead, a small estate adjoining the Institution, and stayed there on many occasions to supervise the work. He visited Redhill four hundred times over the next four years and calculated that this represented a year of his life. He did not stop his visits to Coulsdon and Colchester. In 1853 he again spent Christmas Day at Essex Hall. Leaving there late he reached Shoreditch Station to find that there was no vehicle to carry him home. He walked two miles through a famous snowstorm and a biting north-east wind. He reached home at one o'clock in the morning, shaking with cold, yet took no more harm than a stubborn cold.

Andrew Reed continued his favourite employment until the end of his life, although at times frustrated by ill health. A page in his diary in 1860 demonstrates his level of commitment:

July	**30**	**Earlswood**
	31	**Royal – Putney** (i)
Aug	**1**	**Idiot – Office**
	2	**Fatherless – Office** (ii)
	3	**Colchester**
	4	**Royal – Poultry** (ii)

In 1861 he tendered his resignation as Secretary of the Asylum. He was persuaded to continue on the understanding that he would be relieved of the most onerous duties. He shared the post with John Conolly until his death, at which time Dr. Conolly took on the full responsibility. He continued to attend the elections and the anniversary festivals. During his last days he sent the following message to the Asylum:

> **"My love to them all. Thank them for their letters. Tell them to remember me, and to take care of their sun-dial."** (iii)

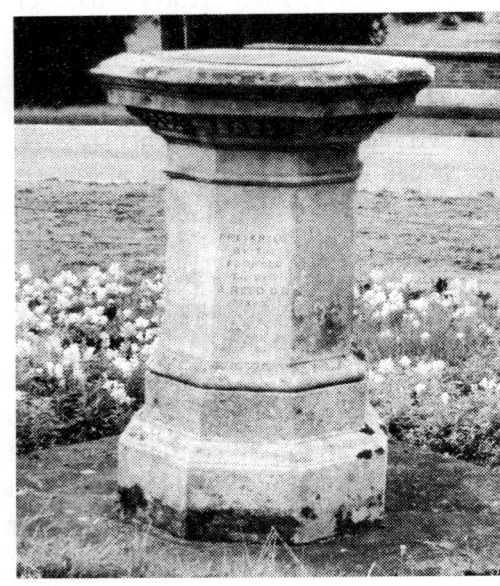

The Sundial presented by Andrew Reed
(Reprinted courtesy of J Street)

When his son, planning his biography, asked him what he would like recorded about his life's work he replied:

> **"I was born yesterday; I shall die tomorrow; and I must not spend today in telling what I have done, but in doing what I may for Him who has done all for me. I sprang from the people; I have lived for the people – the most for the unhappy; and the people, when they shall know it, will not allow me to die out of their loving remembrance"**

> *Andrew Reed D.D.*

(i)	Royal Hospital for Incurables founded by Andrew Reed in 1854
(ii)	The Asylum for the Fatherless founded by Andrew Reed in 1844
(iii)	A gift from Dr. Reed, erected in front of Earlswood.

Andrew Reed died in 1862 in the house that he built adjoining the grounds of Earlswood. A full-length portrait of Andrew Reed, the work of Walter G.R. Browne, was unveiled in July 1875 by the Earl of Shaftesbury in the presence of his son Sir Charles Reed and his wife. It originally hung on the main staircase at Earlswood, but was later moved to its final position in the boardroom. Andrew Reed was also commemorated at Earlswood by a bust on the main staircase.

"The Idiot – A Beam for Mental Defectives" by Eliza Grove

Yet not upon him we gaze,
With cold and despairing eye,
'Tis not decreed that idiot born,
Must a poor idiot die.

Earlswood, the Early Days.

The speed with which both Park House and Essex Hall became over crowded was an indication of the need for a large, purpose built institution to provide security and care for the 'idiot'. As early as 1850 Andrew Reed had recognised this fact and a building fund was launched at the festival dinner in the spring of that year. The Board turned its attention to finding a suitable location within easy reach of London.

An estate comprising 155 acres on Earlswood Common near Reigate was put up for sale in 1850. Due to a misunderstanding the Charity's agent failed to bid for it and it was sold to Mr. Justice Talfourd. On the 4th of November, Andrew Reed wrote to the purchaser explaining the circumstances. Mr Talfourd agreed to transfer the property to the Charity for £15,000, the price that he had paid. He even offered that his own solicitor should complete the arrangements. Mr. Talfourd was to become a life-long supporter of the Asylum at Earlswood.

It took over a year to complete the purchase of the estate. Early in 1852 a competition was launched for architects to submit plans for the new Asylum. The specification was for a building to house 400 residents, approximately 100 infants, 133 boys, 66 girls, 34 women and 66 men. Eight designs were received and the House Committee sought the advice of Mr. Peto and other professional parties to select the best. The first prize of £50 was awarded to Messrs. Kerr and Morgan for a design entitled 'Con Amore'. The second place went to Mr. Moffat for 'Restoration'. The Committee was authorised to make arrangements, on any terms they thought desirable, to secure the use of these plans for the Society. The initial intention to offer Mr. Kerr the post of architect was abandoned when it was discovered that some of his previous work had been unsatisfactory. Instead the post was awarded to Mr. Moffat who was the partner of Sir George Gilbert Scott, architect of the Albert Memorial and St. Pancreas Station. Together with Andrew Reed, Mr. Moffat began visiting institutions to gather information about the best internal layout for the building.

In October 1852 a qualified bailiff was appointed and took up residence in a cottage on the estate. One room within the cottage was set aside for the regular Committee meetings to discuss the management of the grounds and the building process. In late October the Committee met with the Directors of the Brighton Railway to agree the construction of a siding at Earlswood. This was completed in August 1853 and the Traffic Manager for the Railway Company agreed a fixed tariff for the transportation of materials to Earlswood of one penny per mile per ton. The Brighton Railway Company was to become a regular supporter of the institution.

The Committee purchased a further 26 acres adjacent to the Earlswood estate and rented six more. The Board accepted the final plans for the building in March 1853. Tenders were invited for the construction and ten were submitted ranging from £29,400 to £34,600. In May 1853 the Board accepted the lowest bid and building began. In the same month Mr. Sneezum was appointed Clerk of the Works, on a wage of three guineas per week.

The successful tender was one submitted by Mr. Jay, whose company had also been responsible for the building of the Houses of Parliament. However, shortly after it was accepted, he approached the Board explaining that an error in his figures meant that he could not complete the building for the specified amount. He asked to be released from the contract. The Board sought the advice of Mr. Moffat whose own tender had been only £560 more. Mr. Moffat felt that the building could be completed for the original figure and Mr. Jay agreed to abide by this decision. A few months later a contract was completed between Mr. Jay and the owner of the quarry at Gatton Park, Reigate for a supply of stone for the building. The choice of this stone was ultimately to have serious consequences.

Prince Albert, the Prince Consort, took a great interest in the charity from its earliest days. His royal patronage and interest encouraged public support. Consequently, he was invited to lay the foundation stone on Thursday 16th of June 1853. The Board again approached the Brighton Railway Company, this time to request a reduction in fares on behalf of the Society. On the day the foundation stone was laid, the Railway Company ran express trains from London especially for the occasion. Return tickets were 4/- (20p) for first class seats and 3/- (15p) for second class. A special train conveyed Prince Albert to and from the ceremony at a cost of £16 5s. 0d. (£16.25), the cost met by the Railway Company. Two thousand people attended the ceremony. Two laundry baskets were needed to carry away the purses contributed. The donations made on that day alone amounted to £10,000.

Two sureties were required from Mr. Jay and these had been received and accepted by July. A further dispute about the amount of twelve-inch drainage pipe that would be required was eventually settled in December. In January 1854 the contract was finally signed between the

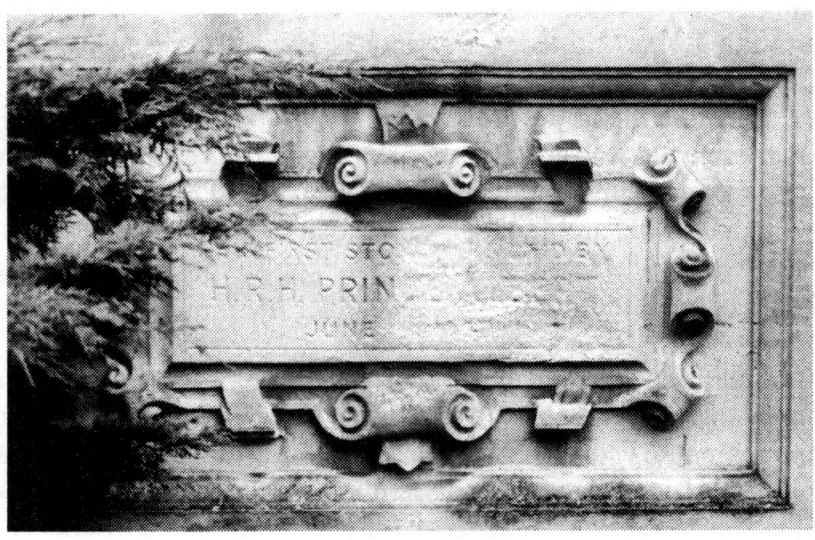

First foundation stone laid 16th June 1853

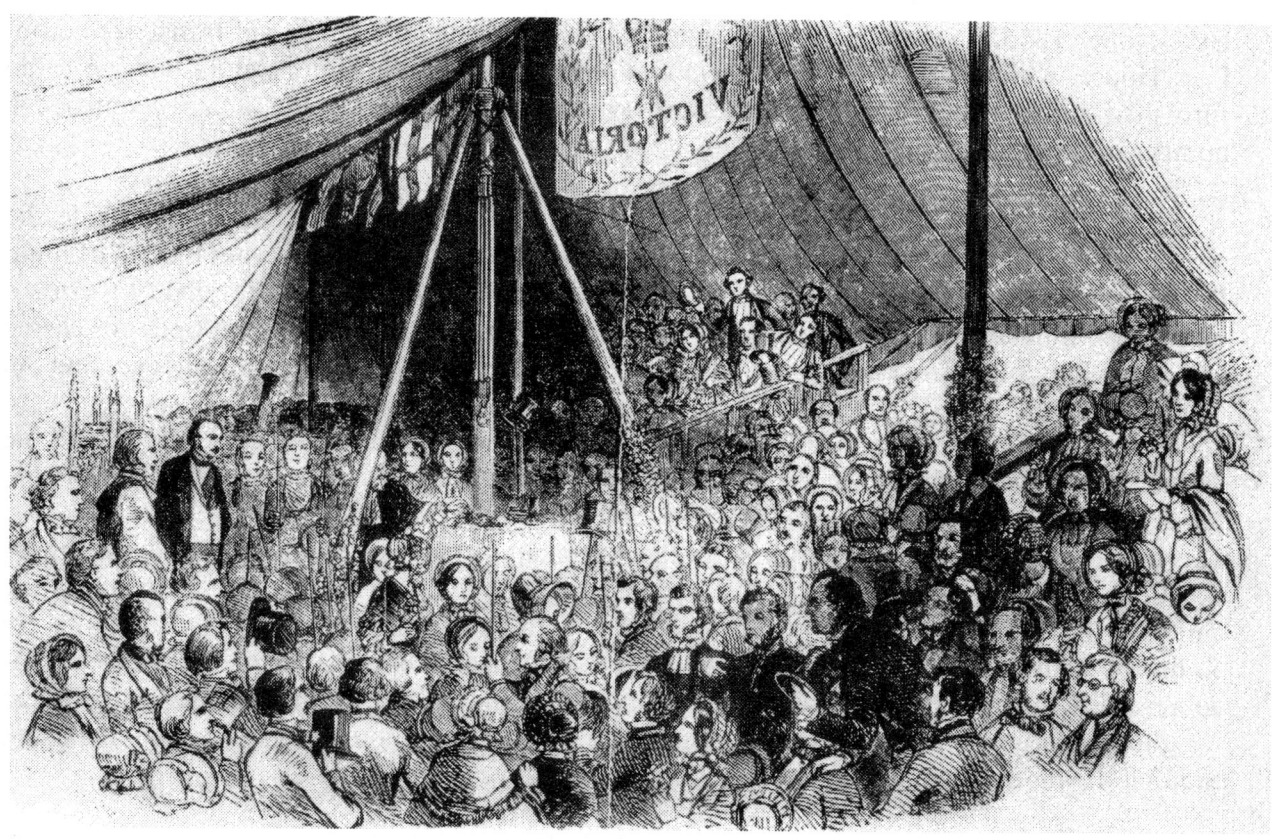

The laying of the first foundation stone

Trustees of the Asylum and the builder and the sum of £509 7s. 5d. (£509.37) was paid to Mr. Jay for the preparation and materials required for the laying of the foundation stone more than six months earlier.

In December 1853 work began on draining and trenching seven acres of land for the kitchen gardens. A road onto the estate was constructed for £30. Unwanted timber on the estate was felled and sold. By September 1854 there were 210 men employed on the project. Also in 1854 the Asylum leased some land on Earlswood Common, together with the Bridge Hotel. This provided accommodation for Board and Committee meetings until the main building was ready for occupation. At that time it reverted to its use as a hotel with public bar.

Funded by public donations or subscriptions, money was never plentiful. Any improvements in the design had to be justified. However, in March 1855 it was agreed that plate glass should be used throughout the building in the interests of comfort and fuel economy. This added a further £1,000 to the cost.

The first residents moved in on the 15th of April 1855. The 'National Asylum for Idiots' was officially opened on the July 5th 1855. Prince Albert once again officiated, this time representing Queen Victoria who had been invited to perform the ceremony. The Prince Consort declared the Asylum open with the words

> **"I hereby declare this Asylum to be open for the care and education of the Idiot and Imbecile for all time to come and may God prosper it."**

The Bishop of Oxford then conducted a religious service.

17

By October 1855 the Asylum already accommodated 70 people. Most had transferred from Park House, which had closed the previous month. Some parts of the Asylum had yet to be furnished and the report of two inspectors for the Commissioners in Lunacy identified a number of problems with the building.

A second visit by the inspectors in February 1856 found the road immediately outside the Asylum to be in a dreadful state. Planks were required to reach the door across the sea of mud. Drainage work costing £60 was required to make the road good. The eastern end of the main range was uninhabitable and the sewage from the institution emptied into an open pit at this end of the building. Limited progress had been made with the kitchens and washhouses and the offices were unfinished. The gasometer and gas fittings were incomplete. The inspectors were concerned about inadequate ventilation in some of the water closets and rooms. They noted the absence of heating in the dining room.

There were two washhouses. The first, in the basement of the main building, was for ordinary washing. It was found to have defective drainage and the fittings were too high for many of the children. The baths could not be accessed from both sides. The water closets (toilets) were equipped with a clever mechanism that caused the flush to operate whenever the seat was depressed. Unfortunately, once again consideration had not been given to the small stature and weight of many of the younger residents. The second washhouse was for foul linen and bedding. It was adjacent to the brook and discharged directly into it.

The inspectors were impressed with the overall design of the building, the arrangement of the apartments and the light, airy, spacious rooms, heated by open fires. The stairs were numerous and convenient, but concern was expressed that they were "not bricked" and the balustrades were dangerously low. The kitchens and dining room they felt to be well situated. The food was plentiful, well cooked and presented.

The number of residents was rising steadily and had reached 123 by the time the inspectors made their visit. Males outnumbered females by almost two to one. The inspectors found a sad lack of furnishings and equipment. The painted bedsteads had lath bottoms that were hard and uncomfortable. One ward, accommodating 31 girls, had only seven drinking cups. The inspectors recommended that the wards should be supplied with cupboards and clothes presses. Future bedsteads were to be polished wood with sacking bottoms. There should be additional washstands, seats and tables, all suitable for children. There were to be mirrors in the wards and lavatories, movable small baths and sufficient crockery. There was also a chronic shortage of staff.

Statutory books were not being kept. The casebooks, which recorded the admission and subsequent progress of each inmate, were still incomplete. It was recommended that all mental and physical defects should be noted and details recorded of treatments tried. The diet table was to be drawn up. The inspectors found the dormitories to be very unpleasant. The mattresses were soaked in urine and stained with ironmould. An urgent recommendation was made that a waking night staff should be appointed to rouse the residents, as necessary, for toileting.

The inspectors found that the girls were clean, tidy and actively employed at their needlework in a spacious and cheerful room. The boys, by contrast, were reported to be untidy and idle, the weather preventing them from engaging in outdoor activity. Pupils did not have the benefit of school exercises. Only two boys were employed in mat making and one was assisting the joiner. They recommended that the roads should be repaired and access provided to the kitchen gardens, where the boys could be provided with work. Some of the boys were put to the breaking of stones for this purpose. Regular exercise was to be taken in the open air and a room made available for the residents to change their dirty shoes on re-entering the building.

Another area of concern was the "turbidity" and brown coloration of the water supply. Staff and residents had been affected by bowel complaints. It was suggested that this problem should be urgently investigated and water filters introduced. The damp and cold conditions naturally found in a building under construction had left a number of residents in bed with catarrh or suffering from chilblains. The inspectors urged that fires be kept alight in the building. Floors were to be buffed rather than washed, wherever possible, to minimise any additional dampness. They also recommended that the temperature should be monitored on every ward.

The inspectors decreed that no more patients should be admitted until the Asylum was completed. They viewed the transfer of residents from Highgate as "precipitate" as the building was "utterly unprepared to receive them...A grave error had been committed."

In 1855 it became necessary for the Board to seek a loan to cover the cost of building at Earlswood. A mortgage was raised for £10,000. A second loan to cover immediate expenses was arranged with the City Bank, secured by members of the Board. By the time the mortgage was finalised in January 1856 it had already become necessary to cease work on part of the building because of a shortage of money. A further £5000 was required in June 1856 as a consequence of the rate of building. Mr. Jay, the contractor, was pressing for settlement and an arbitrator was brought in. He ruled that £5,095.49 must be paid within 14 days and a further £1,500 within three months. The Society was unable to raise another loan and the Board members had to pledge the capital. Mr. Jay, when the situation was explained to him, agreed to wait a little longer for the final settlement.

Appeals were made to ministers sympathetic to the Asylum asking them to preach sermons in favour of the Charity, and advertisements were posted explaining the urgency of the situation and asking for extra donations, or advance payment of charges. In October 1856 a Mr. Huth offered 100 guineas, provided nine others made the same pledge. He paid for the offer to be advertised with immediate success.[i] By the time all payments had been made in 1857 the Society had borrowed £20,000 and the debt was not finally cleared until 1864.

The building was finally completed at the end of 1856. However, the Commissioners in Lunacy were still unhappy with conditions within the Asylum. The water was now described as "dark brown in colour – thick and turbid and quite unfit for drinking purposes." The walls were stained, the floors dirty and the grates had not been cleaned. The dining room was unusable in winter because of the lack of heating. The dormitories were considered to be offensive. The night watch, recommended in the report of the previous February, had not been appointed. The bedding was in a terrible state despite being of good quality. It was stained, one of the mattresses was rotten and in holes and several were wet. During the day the dirty covers were replaced with clean coverlets. This was considered to be a deplorable practice as it gave a false impression to friends and relatives.

Progress was gradually made to remedy these complaints. The closure of Essex Hall in 1858 brought the number of residents to 280. By January 1859 stoves had been installed to warm the building and by June 1861 night superintendents had been appointed. "Pupils of unclean

(i)   Other similar challenges were made in 1860 and 1862.

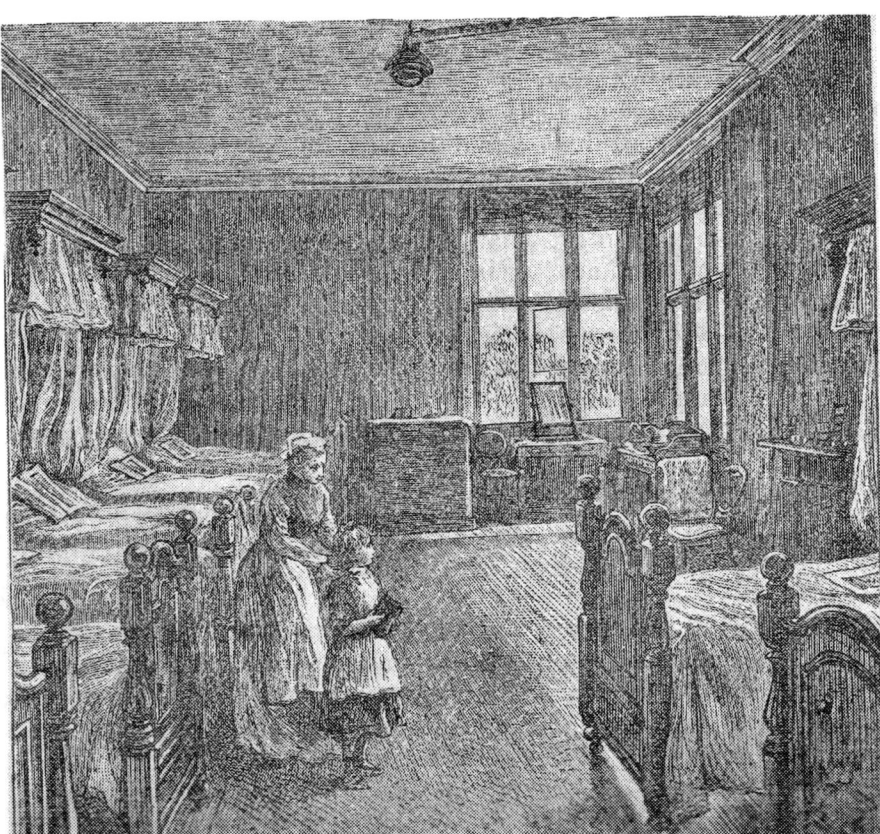

A dormitory at Earlswood

habits" were roused three times per night "by the clapping of hands and upon again being put to bed" they went to sleep immediately "their rest being practically unbroken." An attempt was being made to improve the condition of the drinking water by the boring of an artesian well.

The Asylum was not fully furnished or equipped for a further six years. The total cost for the land, building and furnishings came to £52,000. The Society had accumulated a sizeable debt and no improvements could be considered until this had been paid off. Designed to accommodate 400 residents, the Asylum was only able to offer places to 360 due to insufficient funds.

Daily Life.

The residents of Park House were referred to as the "family" and it was considered to be the duty of the Matron to ensure their well-being. To this end, she regular approached the Board with a list of requests. These ranged from the provision of additional furniture to the removal of unripe fruit from the trees around the building. The boys could not be prevented from picking and eating this, leading to inevitable illness.

The daily routine was quickly established. In December 1848 a formal timetable was set down. The Medical Superintendent supervised the regular exercise sessions. Some children showed remarkable improvement as a result. Dr. Reed recorded the case of one child whom:

> **"...literally began his new life by creeping. As muscular power increased, the little fellow stood, walked, and now he runs. At first he had no notion of holding, but that he might steady himself, he opened the palm of his hand and seized the nearest object. He then learnt to lift a weight, first with one hand,**

6 o'clock	to rise	7 o'clock	to muster
7.15	school exercises	8 o'clock	breakfast
9 o'clock	prayers or exercises in the school or gymnasium		
11 o'clock	recreation	11.30	school exercises
12.30	play	1 o'clock	dinner
2.30	school	4.30	play
6 o'clock	supper	6.30	occupation
7.30	prayer	8 o'clock	bed.

Pupils to rise at 7 a.m. during the winter months – November to February. The period of going to bed may be accommodated to age and season varying from 8 to 9 o'clock.

Wednesday and Saturday afternoons are to be free, the one to receive children's friends, the other for washing and cleansing. The gymnasium exercises are to be taken as much as possible in the open air. The servants and attendants to dine at 2 o'clock. The Master and Assistants having entire charge during that time.

Daily timetable in 1848

afterwards with both; and every week I found him delighted to prove his strength. And with the physical came the intellectual power; and ideas, once formed, were not long in finding some kind of expression."

Reporting progress to the subscribers in 1849 Dr. Reed warned against expectations of immediate results. Nevertheless he felt the Board had seen a reason for optimism.

"Yet it is their privilege to speak of effects partially realised, and in some instances of marked and delightful character. It has been their happiness to observe the eye that had no useful sight, begin to see; the ear to relish sweet sounds; the tongue that was dumb, begin to articulate the language of men; and the limb that was crippled or inert, put forth to useful and active service. In some cases, bad habits have been overcome; power has been created for the care of the person; and both have become subject to mild authority."

The 'Diet Table' or menu laid down in the early days might seem strange to people today, but it was nutritious and demonstrated the desire of the Charity to provide its charges with the best of care. Twenty years later the meals supplied to the residents would be acceptable to a modern diner. The main meal of the day provided four ounces of meat, eight of potato, two ounces of vegetable and six of pudding. For those requiring extra nourishment there was a further ounce of meat and two ounces of pudding. The staple diet was based on boiled or roast beef or mutton, Yorkshire pudding, treacle, rice or bread pudding. Minced meat and mashed potato was provided for those who were known to 'bolt' their food. Most of the foodstuffs were produced on the Institution's own farm.

The residents, when they first arrived at Earlswood, ate on their own ward. When they had acquired reasonable table skills they transferred to the probationary dining room. Having proved their ability they eventually graduated to the main dining room. This beautiful hall had a hammer beam roof and walls half panelled in polished oak. The upper half of the walls, between the windows, had polychrome paintings serving as frames for tablets inscribed with the names of benefactors of the Asylum. Residents experienced a great feeling of pride on the day that they graduated to the main dining room. In 1862 it is recorded that, of the 331 persons resident in Earlswood, 22 were eating in the probationary dining room whilst 170 had skills adequate to admit them to the main hall. By 1880 231 were taking their meals in the main hall, nearly three-quarters were able to use a knife and fork, some a spoon and fork and the remainder a spoon only.

Diet Table   **29 December 1848**

Breakfast
Cocoa, or scotch porridge, or milk and water with bread.

Dinner
5 or 6 ounces of cooked meat with vegetables and bread –occasionally varied with rice, fruit and other puddings.

Supper
Cocoa, porridge or milk and water with plain cake – bread and cheese, bread and butter, or bread and treacle.

The beverage to be water, or table ale, or bitter ale, as the Superintendent may judge to be most suitable. The meat, bread and milk to be of the very best quality.

While care is to be taken that the stomach is not overcharged, the pupils are not to be allowanced by weight or measure; but the Matron and attendants are most carefully to see that all are satisfied, and especially that the food is well cut, well cooked and well masticated.

Soups may be occasionally used, especially in the winter, but they must be meat soups and of most nourishing character. This table is to be accommodated by the Superintendent in such cases which require the aid of medical opinion. Preparation of rice, sago and arrowroot to be made for such cases as may require it – broth, beef tea.

Diet Table from 1848

Mealtimes were carefully orchestrated. Males and females entered the dining room in pairs, by different doors, first the men and boys and then the women and girls. The assembled residents would first sing one verse of a hymn, accompanied by the organ. The individual meals would

---

Table of Cleanliness.   **29 December 1848.**

The pupils are to be washed on rising in the morning and on going to bed at night.
They are to use the bath once a week at least – tepid or cold – unless there should be a special reason to the contrary.
They are to be thoroughly combed twice a week and if needful oftener.
They are to have a change of shirt and stockings twice a week.
Their shoes are to be changed and cleaned every other day.
These regulations are not to interfere with such extra bathings as may be thought to be medically beneficial for any of the patients.
The Matron is to be held responsible for the entire cleanliness of the family, assisted by the nurses and attendants.

Table of cleanliness from 1848.

then be served from heated cabinets. The meals had previously been plated in the kitchen, the portions of each dish carefully weighed to ensure that everyone received their full measure. It is reported that 342 residents could be served in seven minutes by this method. The staff ate once the residents were back in their classes.

Hygiene was considered to be important. In December 1848 the programme of washing and bathing was prescribed. In 1850 a 'manipulator and shampooer' was appointed and the following September it was reported that "the shampooing has a beneficial effect".

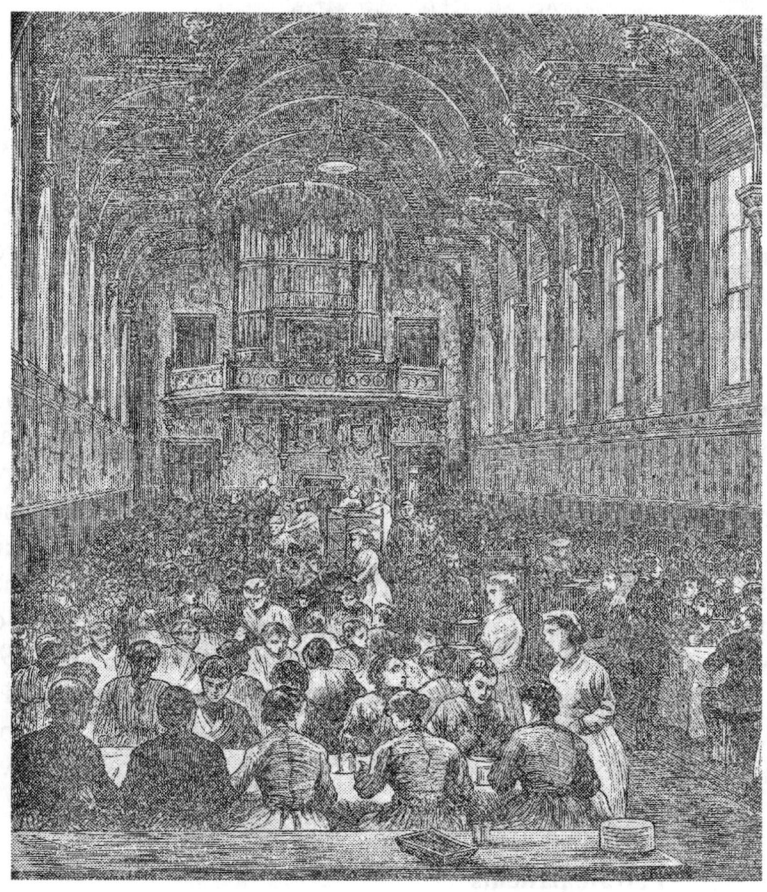

Dining Hall

At Earlswood conditions were generally good. The bathrooms were white tiled and there was ample hot and cold water. Every resident had a cold or tepid bath weekly unless more frequent or warm baths were required for medical reasons. They were washed on rising and before going to bed. Their hair was to be "well combed" twice a week, presumably to eliminate any infestation of lice. Shirts and stockings were changed twice a week and shoes were cleaned regularly.

At Park House relatives and friends were allowed to visit on Wednesday afternoons. They required an admission ticket and only three tickets were allowed in a quarter. Once the Asylum was established at Earlswood, relatives and friends were allowed to visit on Wednesdays and Sundays although they had to notify the medical superintendent at least 24 hours in advance so that "clothes could be drawn from the wardrobe". On normal days the inmates wore work clothes similar to smocks. Sunday best clothes were stored in the wardrobe department and these were available for residents to wear during visits or trips outside the Asylum. The clothes were not personal to the individual but were allocated according to size. This prevented the waste of garments as a child grew.

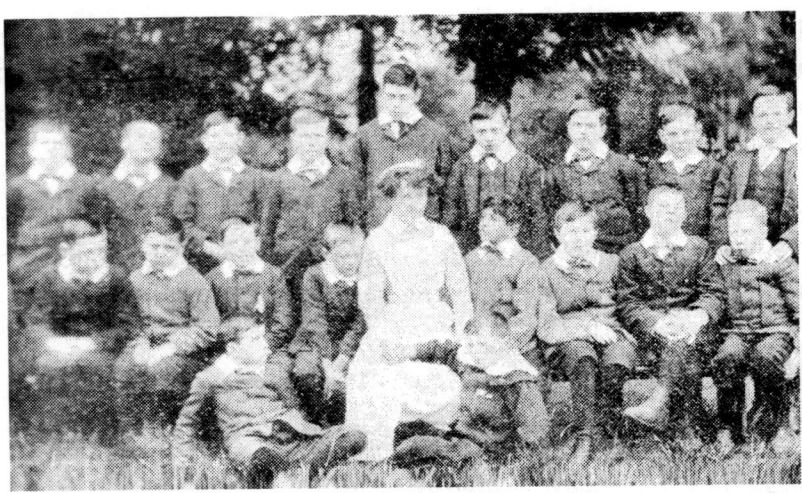

Inmates with a nurse

Patients who were considered to be suitable were allowed to go home on holiday for short periods. They appeared to benefit from this practice. Outings were also arranged on a regular basis and included trips to educational exhibitions and visits to the seaside. In July 1873, 418 of the 569 inmates enjoyed a day visit to Littlehampton.

The residents within the institution were organised into different classes. The individual's placement was decided by factors such as their health, ability or the way that their admission had been funded. This made it simpler to provide the necessary care. 'Payment' or private cases received different treatment from those admitted on part payment or for free. First class patients ate in a private dining room. In 1863 a patient paying 150 guineas per year was provided with a private sitting room and bedroom, together with their own attendant. The accommodation was fitted with superior furnishings and there was carpet on the floor. For 100 guineas the above facilities were shared with only a handful of fellow residents. In 1894 it is recorded that for an extra £24 per annum a resident could eat in a first class room instead of the dining room, £5 per annum would provide a superior bedroom and money could be deposited with the institution to provide pocket money for an inmate. In 1913 the following divisions were recorded:

1st Class	Private patients
2nd Class	'High grade' or more able residents
3rd Class	Small children
4th and 5th Class	Epileptics
6th Class	'Refractory' or less able patients
7th Class	Infirmary.

Those in the lower classes were least aware of their disability. Those in the high grade were conscious of their superiority. Downgrading to a lower class was the most salutary punishment that could be metered out to an offender. They soon attempted by their behaviour to return to their original level. Another form of punishment was confinement in an enclosure where fresh air and exercise could be taken. To be sent there was viewed as a disgrace and residents were careful to avoid misdemeanours.

By 1938 there were nine male classes. The 'high grade' male patients were in a group of 100 whilst there were 30 in the 'refractory' class and these were 'of very mixed ability'. There were eight female divisions, the largest containing 101 residents. The infirmary accepted both sexes. Private patients were still received in 1940. Charges ranged from £175 to £250 although extra comforts could be purchased if required.

Some inmates received particularly special treatment in return for sizeable payments. In the early years one such person was Lord Sefton. He and his private attendant occupied Bridge House and also rented a stable for his pony and cart. The attendant was responsible for Lord Sefton's care and cooked all his meals. Another exclusive resident was the brother of Lord Northcliffe who had two private rooms for his own use.

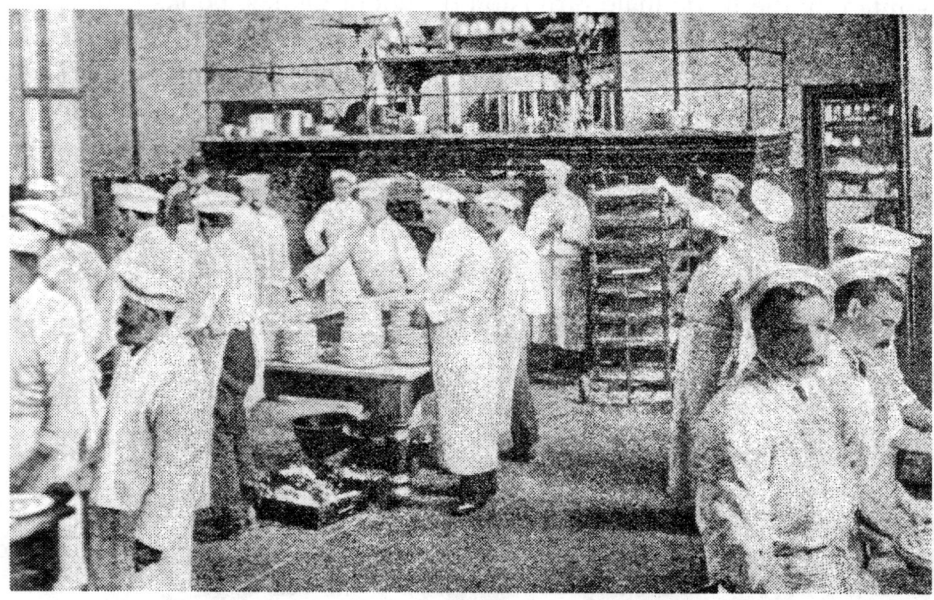

The Kitchen

In 1886 the schoolmistress informed the Board that a number of the residents were now quite infirm, requiring a different form of care. A separate room was set aside for their use, free from the noise and activity of the younger residents.

There were morning and evening services held daily and grace was sung before and after meals. On Sunday the day was occupied with religious services. Morning worship was at 9.15am with bible classes at 11am, although only the boys attended the latter. A further service was held at 3.30pm, with evensong, or 'sacred song service', at 6.30pm. In 1875 about seventy residents went to church in the community, seats being obtained at both church and chapel. A further 370 attended services in the main hall of the Asylum. In the early 1900's nearly sixty per cent of the residents attended at least one church service every Sunday and many attended the daily morning and evening services. Religious instruction was to be "of the simplest character". The Lord's Prayer, the Ten Commandments and the Apostles Creed were felt to be sufficient. Residents could be confirmed if they wished and the annual report of 1961 recorded the confirmation of 13 patients on the 13th of September by the Bishop of Kingston

The children enjoyed various entertainments during the periods of recreation and play. An aviary had been provided, there was a Punch and Judy Show as well as musical events and charades acted with scenery.

The Asylum had its own band and every Wednesday afternoon it would practice in the dining room. . Originally composed of staff members, this changed around 1900 with the formation of a patient band as well. A man's ability to play a musical instrument improved his chance of employment at Earlswood.

Staff generally accompanied inmates on every occasion when they left the asylum although by 1910 there were twelve men who were permitted to venture beyond the boundary without escort. Also in 1910, carriage exercise was provided for three people. Fire drill was practised weekly, with the residents on upper floors exiting by chutes.

Ruth Darwin and W. Rees Thomas, the Commissioners of the Board of Control, noted that the boys played football and cricket whereas there were no organised games available for the girls. They were disappointed by the inadequate provision of indoor games, books and newspapers. They recommended that the children be given the opportunity to join youth organisations such as Guides and Scouts and suggested that the Asylum could operate its own groups. There were further complaints about the lack of gardens and the position of the outdoor area for the 'refractory' class, this being on the north of the building and sunless.

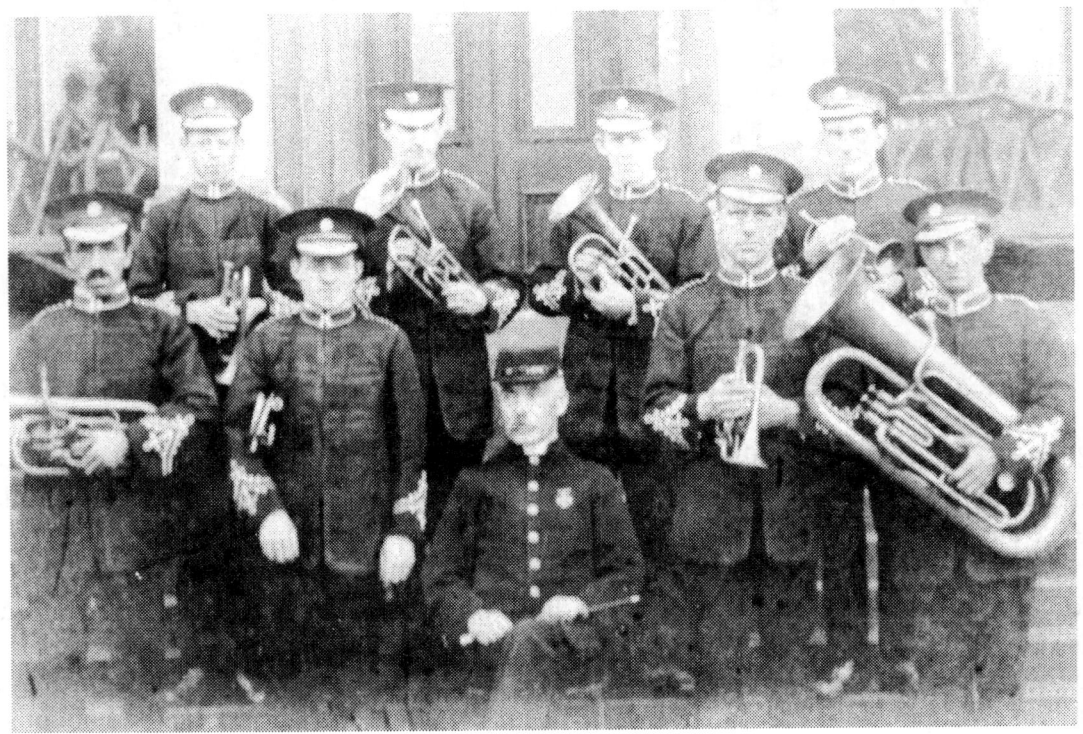

Patients' band

Altogether, Earlswood was a happy place. The magazine *'The Quiver'*, in 1899, recorded that

> **"The sound of laughter in the recreation room, sitting-rooms and playground is almost constant. If it shows the vacant mind, it also bespeaks content."**

The inmates were satisfied with small delights, a new dress or being permitted to listen to the Doctor's watch. Good behaviour was rewarded, in the winter, with the opportunity once a week, to join in games in the recreation room. In summer hard work might be rewarded by an afternoon walk into town or a small amount of pocket money. Most of the residents loved music in particular and it was not unusual for them to request that their birthday be celebrated by the inclusion of a favourite hymn at one of the daily services. *'The Quiver'* described a note, slipped into the hand of the Religious Instructor that read:

> **"Dear Sir, - I wish to ask you in a nice kind way or other, to have two of my hymns on the 5th of February, which is a Saturday. Please have them in the evening – Nos. 590 and 532 – and you may quite expect a nice pocket-book from me. – Your friend, Percy."**

Progress.

After the early problems, conditions started to improve at Earlswood. Things were becoming more organised and life was settling down to a routine. Two storerooms were constructed for groceries and drapery. Linen and ironmongers stores were organised in a waste area of the basement. A large, well-ventilated, well-lit tailors' shop and a cobblers' shop provided employment for 24 and 15 residents respectively.

The scullery was enlarged and all the bathrooms were tiled. A laundry had been constructed and fitted out with the most modern machines for washing, rinsing, wringing and drying clothes. An efficient system was essential as 7000 items were washed weekly. The Asylum no longer needed to send out its washing reducing costs by a half, a saving of £120 per year.

On the ground floor the rooms faced south and provided offices for the Asylum. Above them there were two large dormitories each holding 20 beds. The rest accommodated six or eight. The furnishings were much improved although more ornaments were needed. The varnished bedsteads were enclosed within white dimity curtains and had wicker storage baskets underneath for holding clothes overnight. The residents themselves had manufactured these. Appointment of a night superintendent had significantly reduced the bed wetting and soiling.

The water supply had continued to be a major concern. The new artesian well had reached 840 feet with no sign of water. The main source remained the brook running through the grounds of the Asylum. In 1867, in order to safeguard their supply, the Asylum was forced to petition the House of Lords to prevent Redhill and Warwick Town Water Company diverting the brook. This was of great importance to the Asylum as in 1866 the Asylum had concluded an agreement with Baker and Woodruffe of Tonbridge, Kent for a filtering apparatus for which the company held the patent. The system took less than two months to install and was operational by November 1866. It was capable of purifying 20,000 gallons daily. The Asylum paid £25 per annum rent or royalty but provided the system was used for more than a year Baker and Woodruffe agree that £5 per annum would be returned as a donation to the Asylum. The Asylum had to pay for the installation and the construction of a reservoir. The system seems to have worked and there is reference in future years to the continuation of the annual payment of £25. Considerable investment had been required for the reservoir and for steam engines to pump the water the 1000 feet to the buildings. In addition a tank had been constructed to hold 30,000 gallons of rainwater.

Outside 50 acres had been laid out as pleasure grounds. Eminent nurserymen sent plants for the borders. There were plans for a further 80 acres to be worked as a farm, to provide a substantial proportion of the food required by the institution, as well as employment for a number of the residents.

Visitors were encouraged and many were impressed by what they found. In 1862 the Social Science Congress Excursion visited Earlswood. Entering the front hall they saw the main staircase built in stone and with the bust of Andrew Reed at the top. Above was the central tower rising 90 feet. A wide and airy corridor opened out beyond this and, as the Illustrated London News reported, "the allowance of fresh air to each person is believed to be very much greater than in any other charitable institution in England." Another visitor to Earlswood was Monsieur Mourier, Chief Physician to His Majesty, the Emperor of France. In 1880 M. Tomita, Chargé d'Affaires and several members of a legation visited from Japan where there were plans afoot to build a similar Institution.

A report at the time records how the visitors were greeted by a design of evergreens and flowers with the word 'Welcome' picked out in roses. The walls were decorated with pictures that were the work of the pupils. In a glass case were items of fancy needlework, examples of what could be achieved by the inmates. Also on display were examples of mats, matting, hearthrugs and baskets. A model of a 'man of war'(i) was exhibited in one of the apartments. With the exception of the anchors, this was entirely the work of James Henry Pullen, a resident. It had taken seven years to build.

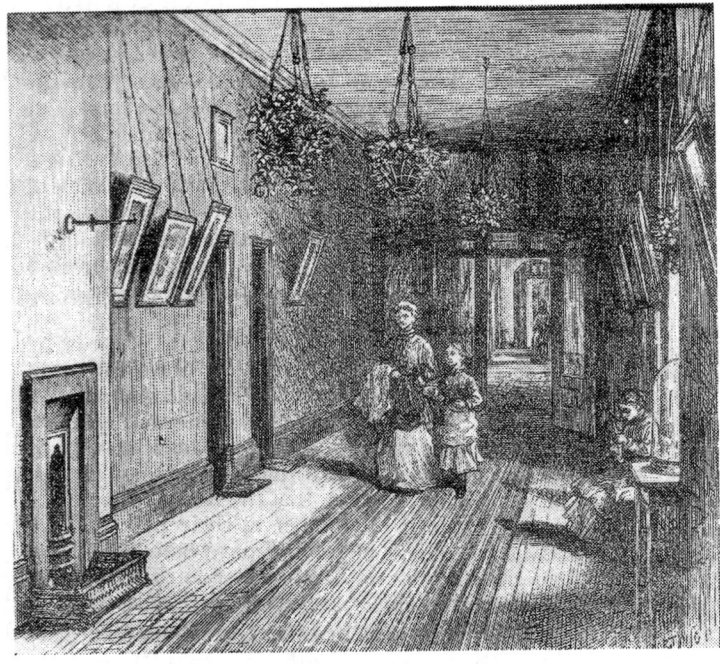

Victoria corridor

Songster birds, in tasteful cages, hung from the ceiling of the main corridor, together with gold and silver fish in glass globes and baskets full of ferns and flowers. Both sides of the corridor were hung with prints and pupils drawings. Friends of the Institution gave pictures and musical instruments.

The total cost of the land, Asylum buildings, well, waterworks and gas works approached £100,000. The gas works did cause some problems in the early days. Henry Boult, Chairman of the Nuisances Removal Committee, wrote to the Asylum under the Nuisance Removal Act for England 1855 regarding the polluting of the local brook, by water and matter from the Asylum Gas Works. The Institution was liable for a fine of £20, together with a penalty of £200, for every day the fouling continued after a period of 24 hours from the serving of the notice. This was an enormous sum for the time.

Enlargement.

The Asylum continued to be successful and the number of residents grew. Within months of the completion of the building there was concern that admission numbers would have to be limited. The Asylum was designed to house 405 cases and already held 377. Forty cases were due to be admitted in the October 1864 elections and only 11 were expected to leave. This would bring the number in the institution to one above the maximum. The medical director

(i)   A warship

28

To the Committee of Management of the Idiot Asylum, Earlswood, near Redhill, Surrey.

Pursuant to a resolution of the Nuisances Removal Committee of the Council of the Borough of Reigate the local authority to execute the Nuisances Removal Act for England 1855 within the said Borough I the undersigned Henry Boult a chairman of the said Committee hereby give you notice that a ditch leading from the premises of the Idiot Asylum at Earlswood within the said Borough into the brook there and also the said brook are fouled by water and matter from the Gas Works on the premises of the said Idiot Asylum. And that you will be liable to forfeit the sum of twenty pounds in addition to a penalty of two hundred pounds for each day during which such fouling shall continue after the expiration of twentyfour hours from the time when this notice shall have been served on you Witness my hand this seventh day of December one thousand eight, hundred and sixtyfour.

Henry Boult

Letter from Reigate Council

29

urged a reduction in the numbers admitted and increases to the rates of payment for private patients. He also recommended that the building be extended as soon as the outstanding debts were cleared. He envisaged wings added to the rear of the building, allowing for the accommodation of between 800 and 1000 persons.

The Society was consolidating and expanding the property. Following Andrew Reed's death his family continued to take an active interest in the running of the Asylum. In addition they agreed to the sale of the estate that he had purchased adjoining Earlswood, to the Asylum, for the favourable price of £2,769-15-6 (£2,769.77). This comprised 14 acres and several cottages. The following year the Society purchased a further six acres of land at the back of the Asylum that it had previously leased. Work continued on the grounds. During 1865 trees and shrubs were planted throughout the gardens, one friend of the institution presented a hundred standard roses. Later, a fine avenue of Wellingtonia trees was planted leading from the front of the Hospital. This was a very appropriate choice as the tree had been first introduced into Britain in 1853, the year in which the Earlswood foundation stone was laid.

In 1865 a new corridor, with additional dormitories, was completed in the east wing over the male section of the Asylum. The boilers, the smithy and the engine house, complete with 12 horse power engine, had been removed to the recently completed laundry building. Later in 1865 Alderman Abbiss, a committee member and staunch supporter of the charity, laid the foundation stone for a new workshop block, to be situated at the east end of the laundry. When this was completed in the summer of 1867 the boys' schoolrooms were moved into the new accommodation and the old classrooms and workshops were converted into additional accommodation allowing a further 24 residents to be admitted.

In 1870 apartments at the east end of the basement were floored and fitted out to provide rooms where the boys could play, especially when the weather was wet. The outside playgrounds had been fenced and a handsome drinking fountain provided by a gift from a benevolent lady. A new basement corridor provided a route through the building to the playrooms and a butcher's shop was situated on its northern side. A newly constructed roadway outside allowed goods to be brought to the basement stores without the heavy carts cutting up the playground in wet weather. A detached mortuary building was constructed and a larger linen room completed.

The increased numbers within the Asylum put a strain on the original facilities and equipment. In 1865 a new oven was built and in 1870 an agreement was signed with Frazer Brothers Railway Iron Works in Bromley for the purchase of new gas and steam cooking equipment, costing £650. The well water was no longer considered fit for consumption and a supply of good quality water was obtained from the Caterham Spring Water Company. An electric alarm system was introduced that linked all the outside and store doors to the Superintendent's house at night. This system allowed the detection of a dishonest night watchman.

At the festival dinner in 1866 plans were finally announced to enlarge the Asylum to house 800 residents. The new building would also provide an opportunity for the classification of patients and the redistribution of accommodation accordingly. The main hall was to be almost doubled in length. On the east and west were planned three storied buildings housing new kitchens, scullery and bake house on the ground floor with female servants quarters above. Covered walkways were to link these buildings to the main block. The top floor would house dormitories for patients and attendants, together with wardrobes, workrooms, lavatories and baths. An organ loft was planned and a fund started towards the purchase of an instrument. It was requested that all payment cases should make a contribution and a total of £155 had been received by the end of the year. The plan also included the construction of a detached infirmary. This was not to be built immediately but later "when funds allowed". The committee was determined to avoid falling into debt again in the process. The estimated cost for the extension was £20,000, so far the building fund contained only a seventh of this figure.

In 1867 the London, Brighton and South Coast Railway opened a station at Earlswood. In 1869 the Asylum purchased four acres of land adjoining the railway, for £600 from the British Land Company. On this the Asylum constructed its own siding, together with sheds, for the delivery and storage of goods transported by rail. This saved the Asylum significant expense and time, as it was no longer necessary to move goods by road from the station to the Institution.

A hotel, with a public bar, was situated on the edge of the Asylum estate. Workmen employed in the construction of the station frequented this. It had proved to be "for a long time a source of great annoyance and anxiety". Earlswood finally bought the property in 1868, together with furniture and fixtures to the value of £211 7s. 6d. (£211.37), from Messr. Nalder and Collyer. It became known as Bridge House and was converted into a dwelling for the Steward and his family. This released further rooms in the main building to provide accommodation for additional residents.

By 1869 the fund for the extension had grown to £10,000, a sufficient amount to allow the Committee to initiate the project. Prince Albert had died in 1861 and Andrew Reed in 1862. H.R.H. Prince Albert Edward, Prince of Wales, later to be Edward VII, consented to lay the foundation stone on the 28th of June. Once again the London, Brighton and South Coast Railway were generous in their support of the Institution. In addition to providing a Royal Train for the Prince and Princess they ran extra trains from London Bridge, Victoria, Kensington and Clapham Junction. They offered reduced priced tickets. A return ticket could be purchased for the price of a single, first class for 4/2 (21 pence) and a second class for 3/2 (16 pence). Special trains also ran from Brighton, costing 5/10 (29 pence) and 4/7 (23 pence) respectively for first and second class return tickets.

There were advertisements in the daily papers three times a week and in the city press. The London Illustrated News charged seven guineas so the entry was only placed once. Posters were placed at thirty railway stations at a cost of ten shillings (50 pence) for every two weeks displayed. There were special tickets for the honorary stewards and the editors of the main papers. Prince and Princess Christian, the Prince and Princess of Teck and the Duke of Cambridge were invited.

At midday the founder's son, Mr. Charles Reed, met the Prince and Princess of Wales at the recently completed Earlswood Station. The platform had been decorated with red and white bunting for the occasion. It was carpeted and choice plants and flowers placed at intervals. The roof was decked with the flags of all nations, the Union Jack and the Danish flag, for the Princess of Wales, displayed prominently. The Prince gave a short address at the station before travelling by carriage to reach the Asylum at 12.15pm. The Medical Superintendent and the Stewards of the Asylum were gathered to greet the Prince and Princess and conduct them to the reception rooms.

All of the residents, with the exception of the nursery cases, were assembled at 10.30am and taken into the grounds for a picnic before returning to the building to watch the ceremony, some from the windows and some outside. At 12.30 a procession was formed and the Prince conducted outside. The address was given, followed by the laying of the stone and the collection of purses of money donated by those in attendance. The Prince was presented with an ivory handled silver trowel bearing the inscription:

> **"Presented**
> **to**
> **H.R.H. the Prince of Wales,**
> **on his laying the first stone**
> **of the**
> **Enlargement of the Asylum for Idiots,**
> **28th June, 1869."**

A glass case was placed in a cavity below the stone. This contained the coins of the realm, a book of the Institution, a list of its members, a list of all the ladies donating purses and of all gentlemen donating at least five guineas, The Prince spread mortar, the stone was lowered on top. Taking the mallet used by his father in 1853 he tapped the stone three times, used the spirit level, also used by The Prince Consort, to check its position and declared it "Well and truly fixed." There was a flourish of trumpets and much cheering.

Following the ceremony the Prince enjoyed a luncheon at the Asylum before leaving at 2.35pm to return to the station. Princess Alexandra was entertained at a private luncheon with her attendants and the wives of committee members, about thirty ladies in all.

After the Royal party had left an incident occurred that was to reach the pages of the local paper. A gala tea took place on the lawns at Earlswood with the food arranged in one of the front rooms of the Asylum. The police were unable to control the confusion arising from overcrowding caused by the 3000 visitors present. A group of the Reigate Volunteers, ancestors of the Territorial Army, had come into the grounds uninvited. Impatient, they forced their way into the room where the food was being prepared and began throwing provisions to their comrades outside. One of the Board members eventually managed to restore order and the Volunteers departed. At 3pm all of the patients were taken down on to the lawns and the summer fete began. An hour later the general public were admitted on payment of one shilling (5 pence). The day finished at 8pm and was deemed a great success. The total number of visitors exceeded 4000 and, despite the behaviour of the Volunteers, "no mishap or casualty of any kind occurred".

The building work came to a temporary halt in the spring of 1871 due to a shortage of funds. The extension to the main hall was not completed until November 1872 and the remainder of the building early in 1873. At this time the Asylum was reorganised to allow more appropriate care of the various classes of patient. The extended hall continued to be used as the main dining room and, in addition, accommodated regular religious services. The Board was forced to borrow money in 1872, 1873 and 1874 to meet expenses. In October 1875 the Board found it necessary to borrow a further £5,900. After the completion of the building, and with the admission of additional payment cases, things improved and by 1877 the Asylum was clear of debt.

On the 5th of August 1876 the Asylum received a visit from a Monsieur Henri Marechal who was greatly impressed by what he saw. He was particularly struck by the use to which one of the large internal courtyards had been put. A roof of iron and glass had been constructed, paid for by a Board member. When the British climate made it unwise to venture out, the residents used the large all-weather space that resulted for their gymnastic sessions. It was also put to use for large assemblies when parents and friends had been invited.

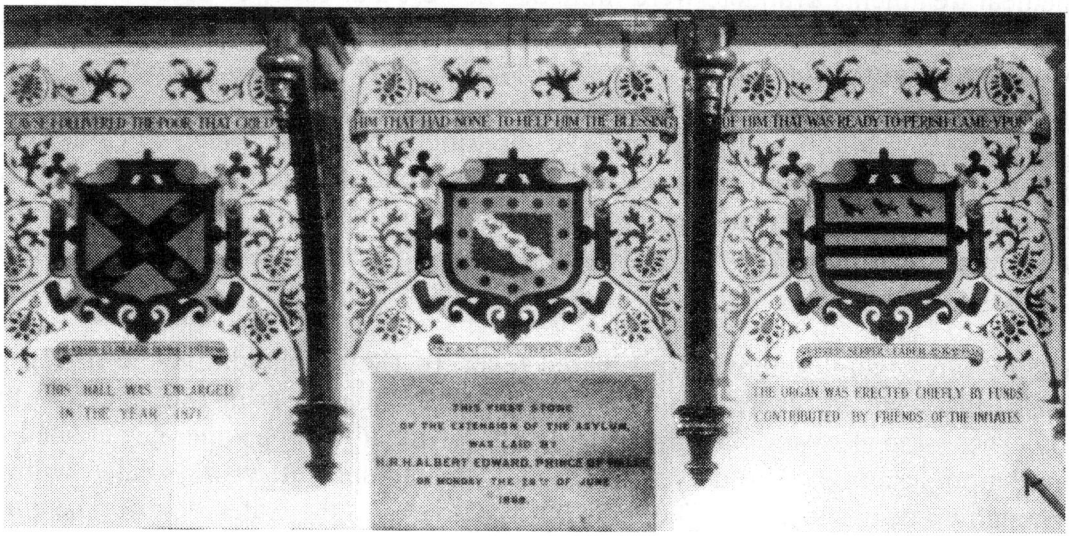

Foundation stone of the first extension
(Reprinted courtesy of J Street)

The growing population within the Asylum was generally healthy but the Commissioners in Lunacy were concerned about the Institution's inability to isolate cases of infection that developed. The staff was already aware of the potential for the development of a serious epidemic. The answer was to construct a detached infirmary. Whilst this plan was put into action and the necessary funding raised, a temporary infirmary was set up in part of the second floor in the north range.

Health.

The residents of Earlswood received the majority of their medical care within the Asylum, a visiting surgeon, assisted by the medical superintendent, even carried out operations. From 1849 a local dentist regularly visited the Asylum.

The first medical emergency faced by the Asylum was an outbreak of scarlet fever in 1852, in which one patient died. Dr. Maxwell and Dr. Reed were authorised to move healthy patients to a different house if the need arose. Scarlet fever was the most common infectious disease at Earlswood in the Victorian period with at least seven outbreaks within the first 50 years resulting in 18 deaths. Over half of these occurred in 1863 during an outbreak which involved 192 cases, 45 amongst the staff. Scarlet fever reached a peak in England as a whole during the 1860s. However, as late as 1912 there was an outbreak in Earlswood that took eight months to stamp out, and in 1925 a further outbreak claimed three lives.

In the early years there were a number of deaths from epilepsy and pulmonary infections, including tuberculosis. Those with epilepsy had originally been excluded from the Asylum. However, this must have changed rapidly and by 1879 there were 150 epileptics in Earlswood. Epidemics of influenza occurred in most years. The cause of death for many clients was given as phthisis, a term describing a wasting disease, perhaps most commonly relating to consumption or tuberculosis. Other regular causes of death were paralysis, apoplexy and chronic infection of the spinal cord.

The medical treatments available were limited. The best that could be offered was good food and hygiene. All reports of this time commented on the cleanliness and order achieved at Earlswood. In August 1866 the inspectors commented on the low level of illness, eight out of 428 residents, "especially during a season when diarrhoea is epidemic and malignant cholera prevails in the metropolis and other parts of the kingdom". There were no cases of cholera during the first fifty years at Earlswood although one child did die whilst on home leave. The cholera epidemic in London left one woman dead, leaving an 'idiot' child. The Board decided to admit the child without election or fee. The members gave their approval and money was soon received in support.

The 1860's saw several outbreaks of typhoid fever. In 1860 typhoid affected fifteen patients and five deaths resulted. There were two deaths from typhoid fever in 1862 and a further four in 1866. The outbreaks were thought to be due to 'effluvia' from a water closet sited close to the ventilation system. In February 1878 31 patients and six staff were isolated with typhoid fever though no deaths resulted. The outbreak was traced to the water supply. The entire area served by the water company was affected. The Asylum cut off its supply and used spring water until the problem was resolved. The new infirmary proved 'invaluable'. Opened in 1878, the building accommodated 48 and was in constant use.

Measles outbreaks were less common but accounted directly for 41 fatalities before 1900. The constitutional weakness remaining in some of those who survived the illness would eventually contribute to many more deaths. There were three major outbreaks in the first 50 years, in 1862-3 there were 120 cases with 19 deaths resulting, and in 1866 another 54 cases and 6 deaths. In 1886 a further epidemic resulted in 16 deaths. Further major outbreaks were to occur in 1917-8, 1938 and 1940, immunisation not being available until 1968.

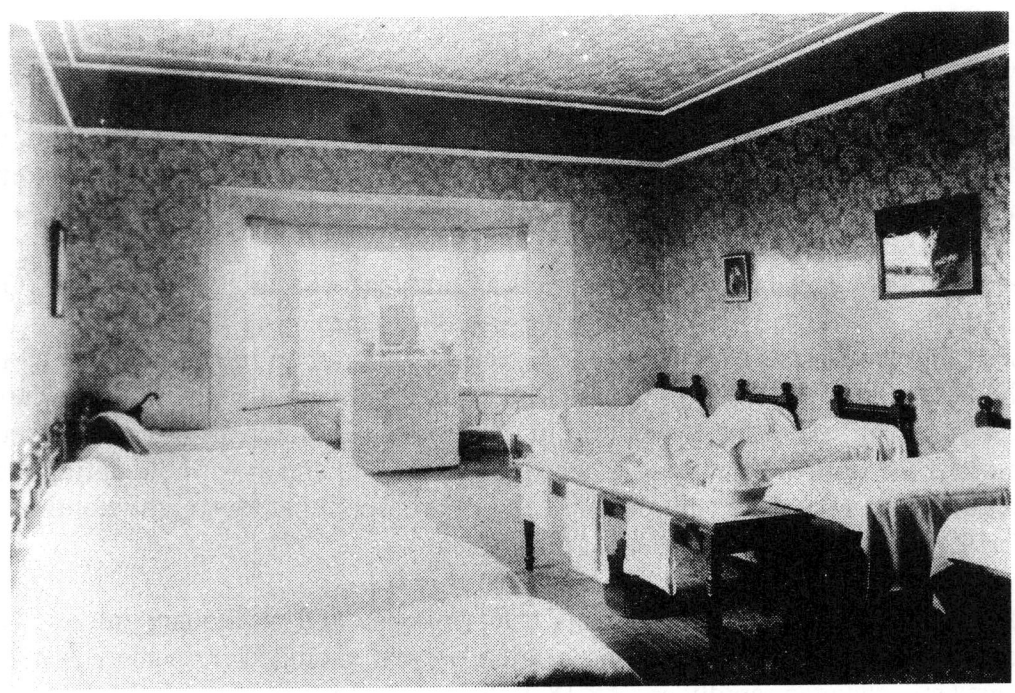

A dormitory

Earlswood was in no way unusual at the time. The mid-nineteenth century was marked by numerous outbreaks of infectious disease within the community as a whole. The spread of infection was still poorly understood and the concentration of the population within the growing towns provided an ideal environment for mass contagion. The new infirmary at Earlswood was soon found to be too small for the demands of the Asylum. The 1880's and 90's saw a number of large epidemics including chicken pox and rubella. Plans were put in place to build a large detached isolation hospital. However, funds were still not available by 1897 and by this time the need for such a building had decreased. As the century drew to a close there was increased understanding of the mechanisms causing epidemics. In August 1890 the Asylum complained to the borough about the proximity of a sewage farm to the Institution. The Town Clerk Alan J Grece responded with a letter in which he pointed out that there had been no increase in morbidity or mortality with a death rate of seven per thousand, the lowest in the borough's history.

The Board advocated all possible preventative measures. Smallpox could be prevented by vaccination. Vaccination of infants was made compulsory in Britain in 1853. Those failing to comply faced a fine of one pound. However, it was not until the serious epidemics of 1871 and 1872 that the law was enforced. At Earlswood all potential candidates had to produce a certificate of vaccination before they could be admitted. Revaccination was also common practice. In 50 years there were only three cases of smallpox reported at Earlswood, the first in 1862, with two more cases in 1876. The latter occasion involved a private patient and their attendant, occupying a separate cottage in the grounds. The low incidence of smallpox recorded at Earlswood contrasted markedly with other closed communities at the time.

The weather in the winter of 1879-80 was particularly severe. However, Earlswood escaped any major infections. The boys' school occupied a separate building requiring the students to brave the weather. In order to avoid this, many of the boys transferred temporarily to the girls' school for the duration of the "big freeze". In order to prevent a recurrence of this problem covered walkways were planned.

At the Annual General Meeting in April 1883 it was reported that the health of the inmates had been generally good. The death rate in the hospital was 4.6% of the total bed number or 5.1% of the average occupancy. Sixteen of the fatalities were due to tuberculosis or epilepsy. There had also been some cases of diphtheria. Diphtheria was common in England at the time but Earlswood escaped the worst of the disease. There were several small outbreaks including one in 1883 that claimed the life of a six year old girl. In 1886-7 the last outbreak of the century, and the most serious, affected 72 people and resulted in 13 deaths. In 1927 the summer fete was cancelled due to several cases of the disease, one fatal.

During major restoration work that occurred at Earlswood early in the twentieth century there was an increase in the number of deaths with 29 in 1904 alone, many from tuberculosis, pneumonia and lung complaints. It was impossible to remove all of the residents during the building work and the dust and other inconveniences inevitable during major reconstruction took their toll of those with a weak constitution. Temporary accommodation was found for 120 of the epileptic cases, including the use of a "commodious iron building".

The mortality rate in 1908 was 4%. There were 35 deaths between May 1907 and May 1909, thirteen from tuberculosis and 3 from senile decay. The average age at death was 42 years in males and 32 in females. The Commissioner in Lunacy recommended open air treatment for the consumptive. As a result balconies were included in the rebuilding of the north east wing. Despite this, in 1917 consumption was still the cause of 30% of deaths in the hospital

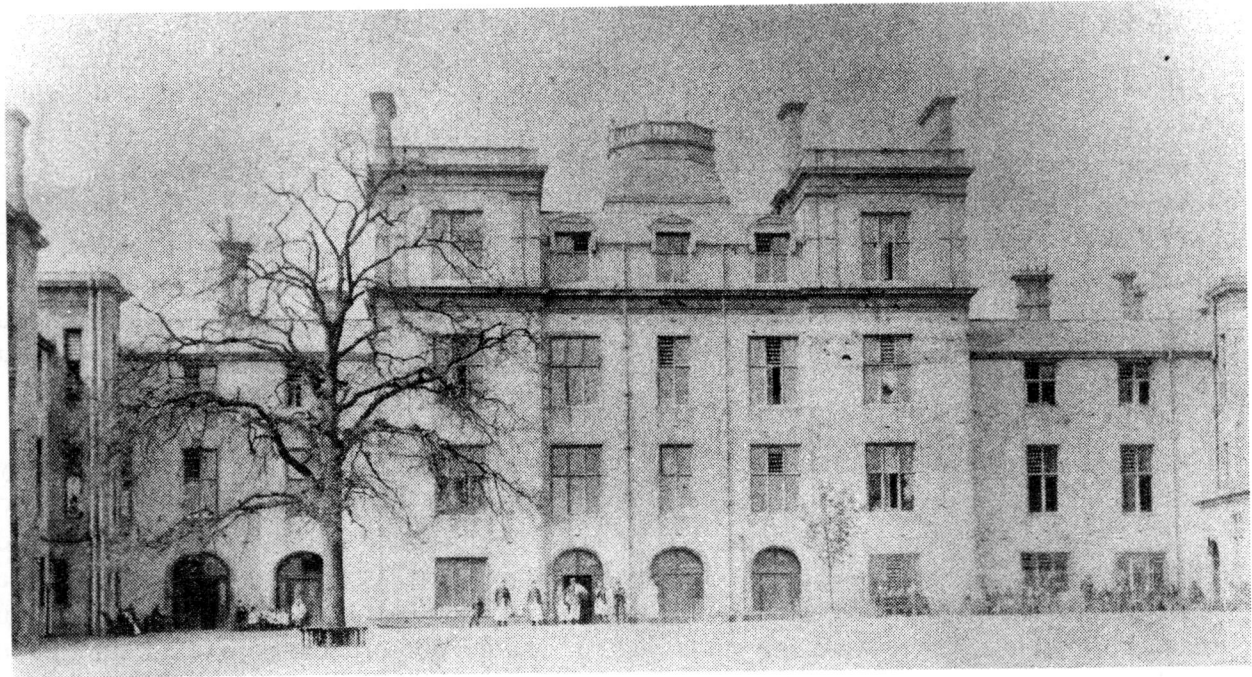

An early photograph of Earlswood

The Royal Commission of 1908 praised the Asylum for the progress that had been made. Measles epidemics were now almost unknown. Previously there had been a whole ward of 'consumptives', this was no longer the case. The infirmary housed mainly those who were physically disabled or chronically sick. Those with acute illness were cared for on their own wards, as a rule, and attended the infirmary only to see the doctor or for treatment.

The *'Charity Record'* in April 1910 recorded that there had been nine deaths in the previous five months. All had been from natural causes and the level of care had been high, one indicator was the lack of any pressure sores. An inquest had taken place into a death from a strangulated hernia but there had been no blame placed on the care offered by the Asylum. A large proportion of the deaths had been from tuberculosis. There were only eleven patients in bed at the time due to illness.

Epidemics did still occur. The New Year celebrations in 1912 had to be called off due to an outbreak of scarlet fever. Initially, there were only about twelve cases, all of mild form and all isolated. However, it was to take eight months before the disease was eradicated. July 1913 saw an epidemic of measles with several children developing pneumonia, though fortunately there were no deaths. A severe epidemic of scarlet fever struck in 1916, a time when staffing levels were reduced due to the number of men who had joined the armed forces and were fighting in the war. Forty five residents and a number of staff were affected. Bridge House was opened up and converted into a makeshift infirmary with three staff to care for all the invalids.

In 1917 there was an outbreak of influenza and at the end of the year a large-scale epidemic of measles. Over a period of several months there were 144 cases in total. A further outbreak of scarlet fever occurred in January 1925, affecting 32 residents with three deaths resulting. In January 1937 there was an epidemic of influenza affecting 70 males and 64 females. In 1938 a further mild epidemic of influenza occurred. However it was followed by a severe epidemic of measles, complicated by bronchopneumonia in many cases, with 85 residents affected, 52 of them children. There were seven deaths as a result. In early 1939 there were 56 cases of influenza, three complicated with bronchopneumonia and one death ensued. The most modern treatments were used within the Asylum. In this case sulphanamide was used to control the infection with good results.

In March 1940 there was an outbreak of rubella, followed by an epidemic of severe measles. Ten of the younger children developed pneumonic complications, with four deaths resulting. Rationing had been introduced by the end of 1941. This did not cause any problems for the lower grade patients. The higher grade residents did lose a few pounds but this was insufficient to be of concern. July saw an outbreak of chickenpox with fourteen cases recorded. There were also 2 major operations carried out in the year by Mr. F. Curtis, F.R.C.S. Nineteen forty-two saw an outbreak of mumps that lasted for the whole of the second half of the year. Up to ten children were in the infirmary at any one time but all recovered successfully. In the summer of 1943 there was an outbreak of infectious hepatitis. In the autumn there were seven cases of scarlet fever and five of chicken pox. Two major operations took place.

Despite the discovery of antibiotics there were two cases of tuberculosis in 1945, one of which proved fatal. Three cases of mumps occurred in the following year. Seventeen people were diagnosed with chicken pox in July 1946 and in September there was an outbreak of gastric influenza affecting 48 people. There was one death from TB. The health of the residents was carefully monitored and a general reduction in weight was put down to the rationing of fats during and following the war. In 1947 21 patients died due to infection and there was concern about the high incidence and the apparent reduction in resistance to infectious diseases. In March there were 28 cases of influenza and in August there were 15 cases of rubella. Five people died from TB in the year. Things then began to improve with a reduction in infectious disease. In November 1949 there were three cases of infantile paralysis. Between July and December 1949 there were 14 deaths, with an average age of 43 years.

In 1950 there were signs that the effects of rationing were lessening with an average increase of three pounds in the weight of the residents. However, epidemics were still a problem. Thirty-six children contracted chickenpox. This epidemic was followed by an outbreak of a particularly virulent strain of measles. Penicillin and sulphonamide was used but for the seriously ill patients another remedy was reported to be a life-saver. Thirty millilitres of blood taken from convalescent patients was injected into the muscle of the ill patient on each of three consecutive days, presumably to stimulate their own body's ability to produce antibodies.

March 1951 saw another epidemic of influenza. In 1952 there were no epidemics or infectious disease. Four hundred patients took advantage of the service recently introduced in Britain, the mobile mass X-ray unit. March and April 1956 saw a sudden outbreak of Sonne Dysentry, with 120 cases of severe diarrhoea. Treatment with antibiotics was effective but the symptoms were very unpleasant. The mass X-ray unit picked up two cases of tuberculosis in that year. Nineteen fifty-seven was not a good year with a total of 18 deaths, five during an epidemic of Asian flu. However no new cases of TB were diagnosed in that year or the next although 1958 saw epidemics of chickenpox and whooping cough. An epidemic of influenza struck the hospital in October and November 1960 with over 200 cases. The mass X-ray unit spent two days at the hospital but fortunately found no cases of TB.

Earlswood continued to try to prevent infections as it had always done. An epidemic of smallpox in Britain in 1962 led to the vaccination of all patients aged 60 or less. This, however, did nothing to prevent a short epidemic of Sonne Dysentry in March of that year, or an outbreak of rubella on the female wards through September and October. Outbreaks of jaundice and dysentery occurred in 1968.

Some groups of clients were particular prone to health problems. Those with epilepsy were at particular risk. The infirmary housed the worst cases including two or three suffering from paralysis. Many people died from epilepsy, 15 in 1880 alone. A report in the British Medical Journal in 1917 recorded that 30% of deaths were from tuberculosis and 20% from epilepsy. Thirty-nine residents died in that year, including five patients who had been in Earlswood for 60, 58, 50, 49 and 43 years respectively. Those with Downs Syndrome, in the early part of the 20th century, rarely lived much beyond twenty years. However, all efforts were made to improve their prognosis and their quality of life. Medical treatment was not only offered within the Asylum. The medical superintendent in 1910 had noticed that the patients with Downs Syndrome were prone to an unusual form of cataract. An eminent ophthalmic surgeon from Guy's Hospital carried out special investigations.

Despite all efforts the life expectancy of those with a Learning Disability was lower than that of the rest of the population. The death rate reached 10% in 1863, the year of the most serious scarlet fever epidemic. Health improved as the nineteenth century came to a close. However, the average age at death in 1937 was still only 38 years. Earlswood at the time housed 67 residents with Downs Syndrome and 72 with epilepsy.

Period	Average National Rate	Average Asylum Rate
1870-2	2.2%	5.7%
1880-2	2.0%	4.6%
1890-2	2.0%	2.8%

Comparison of the death rate in Earlswood with the national average.

For 118 years the health of the residents of Earlswood was the responsibility of the Hospital's medical staff. However, this changed on the first of November 1973 when their physical care transferred to a G.P. practice. This system remained in place until Earlswood closed in 1997. Daily surgeries were held at Royal Earlswood. The G.P. on duty visited those unable to attend the surgery on their home.

The Admission System.

Until the third decade of the 19th century medical treatment was generally only available to those who could afford to pay for it. In about 1828 a system was introduced in Britain that allowed poorer people to obtain medical treatment by applying to a prominent person, such as a Member of Parliament, for a 'ticket' or by obtaining votes. In the early days at Earlswood, most applicants sought election and, if successful, were received gratuitously. Of the first 2000 admissions over half paid nothing. The subscribers to the Charity were entitled to votes in return for their donation. A subscription of one guinea (£1.05) purchased two votes at each of the elections held on the last Thursday in April and October each year or alternatively four votes in one election only. A single gift of five guineas entitled the member to one vote per election, for life. Two guineas annually, or twenty guineas as a single donation, entitled a member to become a governor and, if male, to be elected to the Board of Management. Firms and Corporations that contributed five guineas were allowed two votes annually for a period of twenty-one years.

Suitable candidates could also be admitted if their relatives or friends could pay the amount required. A 'payment' place could be obtained for the sum of twenty-five to fifty guineas per year. Those paying the higher amount were known as 'Parlour Pupils' and were eligible for special privileges. In August 1848 a particular room was reserved for their use. In 1873 the standard charge was £45 a year, and the highest sum paid for any patient was £220 per annum. In 1881 there were one hundred and thirty-seven payment cases and six of them had their own private rooms and attendants. In 1892 the lowest sum for separate accommodation was £150 per annum. By 1899 the cost of the standard payment case had increased to about sixty-five guineas. In 1911 payment ranged up to £500 or more, whilst special cases under 16 years of age could be admitted for a guinea per week. Entry by payment was allowed at any time of the year.

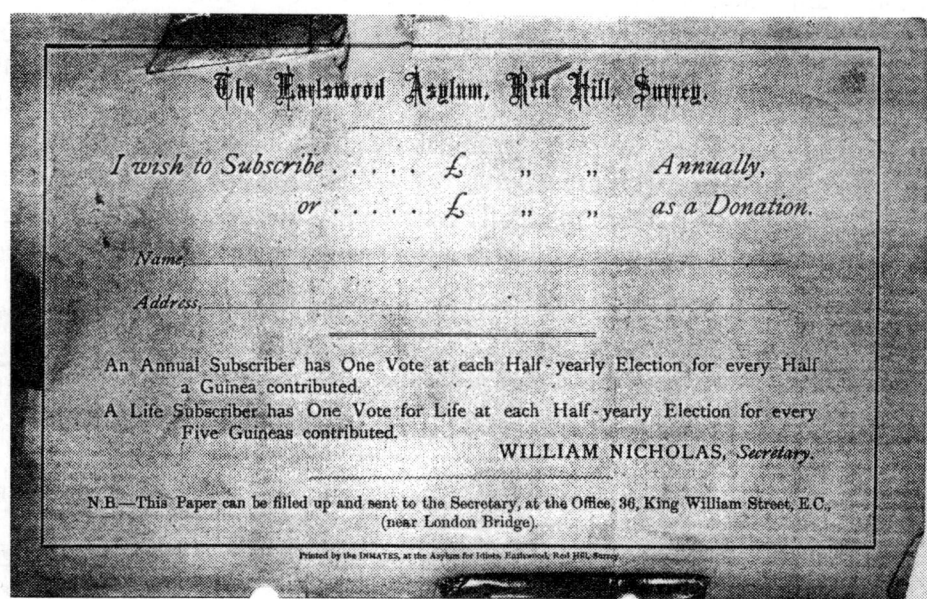

Subscription form

Ability to pay did not guarantee admission. Many cases were refused on the grounds that they were unfit. Reasons given included age, hopelessness, epilepsy, badness, insanity or a combination of the above. In later years epileptics were admitted. By 1881 two hundred of the 561 patients suffered from convulsions. Lunacy was always a bar to entry and if a candidate was found to be 'insane' after admission their immediate removal was required. Uncontrollable violence would also result in the family being requested to remove the patient. Four patients were removed in the first year at Park House, and a further three a year later. A transfer to Northampton Lunatic Asylum was arranged for one girl who was "decidedly insane". Later several children were removed as a result of the inability of the family to keep up payments. Very few children were removed at the request of their family or friends.

If a person was to be admitted to the Asylum their family or friends were first required to apply to the Society offices. Satisfactory answers to certain questions would ensure the candidates suitability for admission. The aim was to open the Asylum to anyone who had need of the care it had to offer.

"...the proper object of the Institution be the Idiot, without regard to sex or place – that such persons as are destitute of means, shall be placed on the foundation, by the open election of the subscribers; while such as have means, shall be supplied with the advantages of the Asylum on moderate payments to be regulated by the Board of Direction, and independent of the Electors."

However, very quickly the position regarding pauper cases was qualified;

> **"That the mere pauper case is not eligible for this Institution but that if it should appear that a case is likely to derive benefit from the treatment adopted, temporary relief from the Parish shall not be an absolute bar to admission."**

Every applicant was investigated financially and medically and needed the backing of at least two respectable people who agreed to remove the patient if required by the Society, and certainly at the end of the term. This first hurdle overcome, the next step was to persuade the subscribers that their votes should be cast in favour of your relative or friend. The Society printed a list of all subscribers each year but it was beyond the ability of many families to orchestrate an election 'campaign'. There were professional canvassers who would undertake this task for a fee. Other families would place adverts in newspapers or approach the guilds, trade organisations or ministers of the Church asking them to use their influence on behalf of their loved ones. Any minister who preached on behalf of the Charity, and any executor paying a legacy of £100 or more, would automatically receive life membership and voting rights. They would also be able to approach other members whose votes were not yet committed.

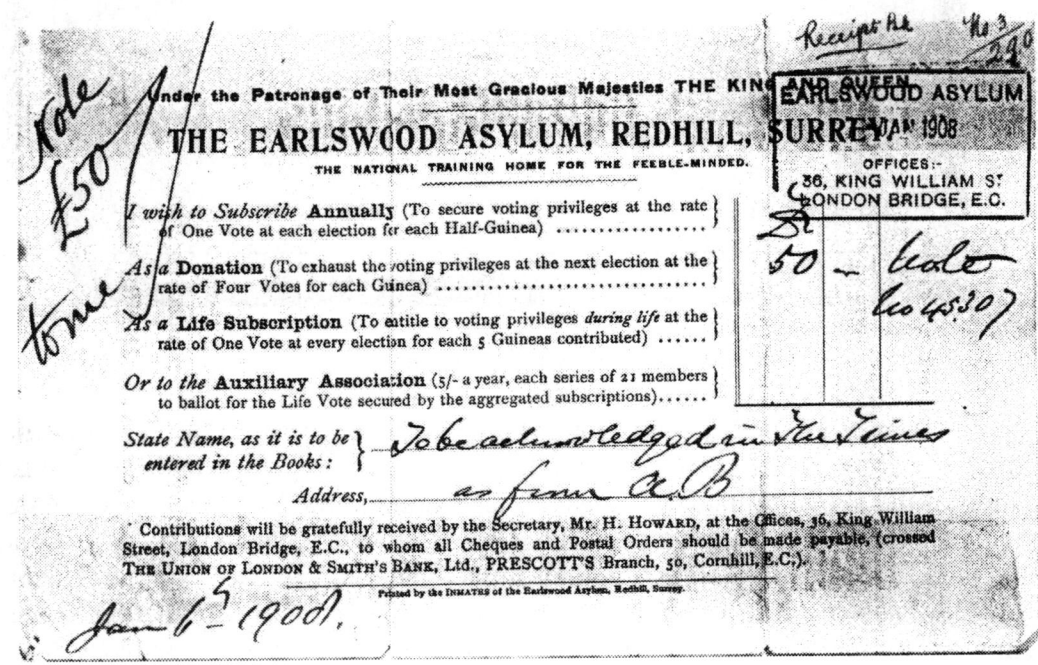

Subscription form from 1908

The first election was unique, taking place on the 21st of January 1848. This was before the acquisition of Park House but the Board of Management wished to avoid any delay between the opening of the Institution and the admission of the first patients. Ten cases were elected on that day and a total of 17 children were admitted on the 26th of April 1848. A further election took place the day after the Asylum opened. Six children were successful from the 75 who applied for election. The successful candidates polled between 727 and 1070 votes. Ten children were elected the following October and again in April, with a further five gaining payment places on each occasion. By this time serious overcrowding was a problem only partially alleviated by the opening of Essex Hall.

Two cases from the same family could not stand for election at the same time, and not more than two members of one family could be received by election. The candidates gaining the highest count would be successful. It was generally necessary to obtain a minimum of 600 votes. If a candidate was unsuccessful at one election, votes could be 'banked' and accrued over a total of three elections. This was increased in 1864 to six. If admission had not been obtained by this time the individual would be ineligible for further elections. Some candidates obtained far more votes than the minimum required. In 1882 the candidate polling the highest number of votes, 1755, was the son of a native schoolmistress from Jamaica. No restrictions were put on race or creed. There are records of children admitted from New Zealand, Hungary, Germany and Prussia.

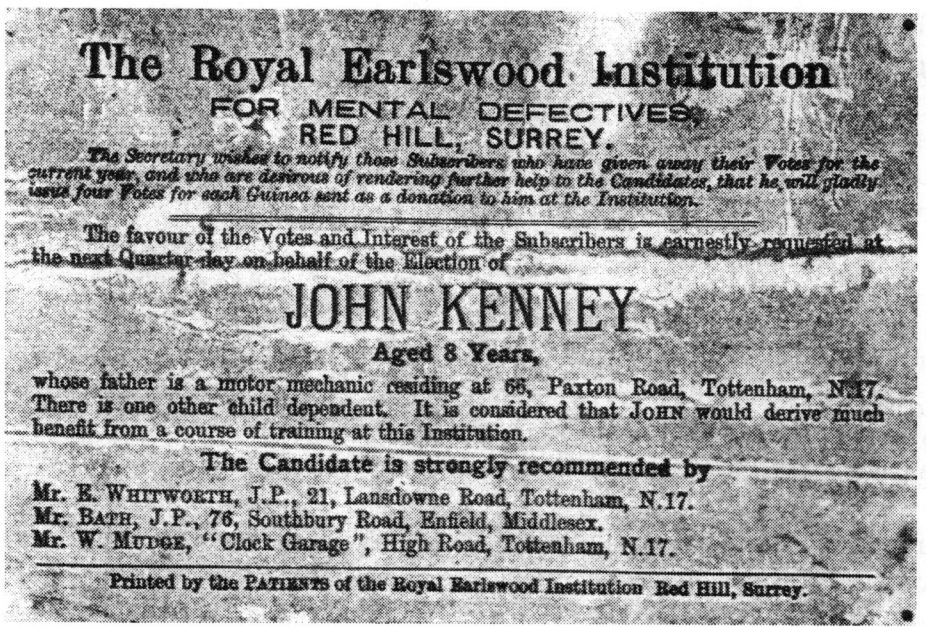

Card distributed to subscribers to canvass votes

The number who could be elected at the meetings in April and October would depend on the vacancies in the Asylum. During the early years at Earlswood it was generally possible to admit between 20 and 40 at each election. A limit on admissions due to lack of space was rectified by the completion of the extension. A shortage of funds in the last years of the century also had an impact on admissions, increasing the number of votes required to about 750. In 1882, at the Annual Festival, it was reported that Earlswood could accommodate 200 additional children but for a lack of funds. This was the result of a reduction in subscriptions and donations caused by public apathy or perhaps other issues gaining public sympathy, such as the victims of the Boar War. The highest number of admissions at any one election was in April 1887 when 50 patients were elected, in celebration of Queen Victoria's Golden Jubilee.

In the early years the elections were held at the London Tavern in Bishopsgate Street, London. This renowned eating place and venue for public meetings was featured in Charles Dickens' novel 'Nicholas Nickleby'. By April 1880 the Annual General Court and Election was being held at the City Terminal Hotel in Cannon Street. Polling took place between noon and 2 p.m. Candidates were not required to attend the election as the Board felt this would be too stressful for them. Polling papers were available in advance to allow for postal votes. The paper listed the name and brief details of each person and, those for whom the election represented their sixth and final chance were indicated with a star. The father's occupation was given and there were representatives of all the trades and crafts, railways workers, labourers and servants. At the spring election in 1883 the Archbishop of Canterbury agreed to become a president of the charity.

Initially there was no age limit to admission although it was expected that children would make up the majority of cases presented for election. By the end of 1852 only those below 20 years of age were eligible. This was reduced to twelve years before being increased to sixteen by 1865. In 1883 the limit was removed. The Board had the discretion to admit those above the age limit and there was apparently no restriction for those who were able to pay. Generally children were not admitted below the age of five. However, between 1848 and 1892, age at admission ranged from three to 54 years.

The purpose of the Charity from the beginning was not merely to house the 'idiot' but to educate him. Those who were considered incapable of improvement were initially not eligible for election. However, the policy was not strictly applied. The Board recognised three classes.

Class 1.'Very improvable cases'
Class 2.'Less improvable cases'
Class 3.'Scarcely or wholly unimprovable cases'

In 1866 the Medical Officers examined the most recent intake of elected cases and found 25% in class 1, 50% in class 2 and 25% in class 3. This shows that the Charity was not favouring the very 'improvable' cases at the expense of the severely afflicted. The Board hoped that class 3 would eventually be housed in a separate hospital, being aware of the difficulty faced by families with a severely disabled member. By 1883 the Board accepted that the truly helpless case was as much in need of care as the more able.

Initially, admission was for a period of five years although early discharge was possible if it was considered that sufficient improvement had been made. Residents could also be discharged 'on licence'. This meant that they were able to return during the remainder of their term if their improvement was not maintained following discharge. At the end of the five years, re-election could be sought if a case showed promise. Some residents improved sufficiently to remain in the Institution as servants.

The five year limit originally applied to election and payment cases alike. However, in 1852, after the decision had been taken to build Earlswood, a case was accepted for life on payment of £500. By April 1857 there were four life cases out of a total of 168 residents. A decision was made to allow those seeking re-election to apply for life. In April 1862 five case were elected for life, achieving between 1400 and 2200 votes, and 20 were admitted for the standard period requiring only about a third of this total. In October 1863 there were 117 candidates for five years and 15 for life places. By 1865 there was one life case elected for every five ordinary cases. Between 1853 and 1886 only 18% of cases stayed more than ten years, 92% were admitted once, seven percent were re-elected, one percent were re-elected on two or more occasions. Most spent between six months and two years at home between admissions. Later on re-admission became more common. By the 1860s there were over 10,000 general and life voters giving Earlswood the second largest subscriber list of any UK charity.

Initially patients were eligible for admission only by payment or election but in April 1876 a system of part payment was introduced. This provided an additional source of income from those who could not afford to pay for total care but who could make a contribution. In 1880 the funds raised this way contributed about £1,500 to the running of the Asylum. The Mental Deficiency Act passes in 1913 resulted in more people opting for part payment, costing 15 guineas per year. Election and part payment cases received the same treatment within the Hospital whilst payment cases were provided with superior accommodation and meals.

In 1902 it was decided to increase the standard term of admission to seven years. The five year term was felt to be too short for the necessary training to be given. It also put a great deal of strain on parents and friends who had to canvas for votes for re-election. One child wrote to his friends,

"It will be soon time to get me in again for another five years. I hope that it will be alright; I like Earlswood."

This was felt to favour rival institutions such as the Metropolitan Asylum Board. It was proposed to make part payment admission for seven years and non-payment for only five years to encourage relatives to choose the former option if it was at all possible. The result was a reduction in the number of cases that could be elected on each occasion. In 1905 twelve males and eight females were admitted by election, a further nine males and one female by election and part payment whilst 12 males and three females were admitted by payment alone. In April 1906 only 25 were elected out of 76 candidates, in October of the same year 73 applied for 20 places. Only 20 to 25 places were available at each election during the years that followed. In October 1915 the number elected dropped to 12 out of the 32 who applied. Meanwhile census data showed that there were 150,000 'feeble-minded' people in England and Wales.

The Board decided that special conditions for admission should apply at the elections in October 1911 and in 1912. The *'Charity Record'* published on May 4th 1912 reported that 12 cases, who had previously been unsuccessful in four or more elections, had been admitted in October 1911 in memory of Edward VII. Despite problems in funding all the cases requesting admission, the *'Morning Post'* of the 24th of April 1912 carried the announcement that the child of any missing crew member of the 'Titanic' would, if eligible, be admitted for seven years free and without election. There is no record that any such case occurred.

In 1914 twelve part-payment and four ordinary applicants were elected. In 1917 the electoral system was altered. It was no longer the candidates with the maximum votes who were admitted but those with a combination of a specific number of votes and the ability to make a financial contribution. A person with 500 votes and 40 guineas in partial payment would be better placed that someone with 1000 votes but only 15 guineas. This change was unpopular in some quarters.

In 1940 the number of votes required to admit a person was decreased by 30% to reduce the cost and effort involved in canvassing during the war. However, vacancies were advertised for payment cases. In 1946 the standard term was again decreased to five years because of a shortage of accommodation. At this time the minimum charge for a payment case was £150.

Only two years later the Asylum ceased to be a private institution and was 'absorbed' into the new National Health Service. This resulted in changes to the way admissions occurred. The voting system was abolished. From 1951 children of all ages were eligible for admission, previously it had generally been limited to those over five. In 1952 the first short-term admissions occurred as respite care was introduced.

The system of elections was perhaps the only way to control admissions as the demand for places at the Asylum far outstripped supply. In 1862 one hundred and seventy one people applied for the 30 available places. Things were no better in 1867 when only 30 candidates were successful out of the 216 who applied. In addition 60 payment cases were awaiting admission. By 1874 things had reached crisis point with only four candidates elected, two for standard term and two for life, out of a total of 227 approved candidates. However, as the maximum quota of life cases allowed at the time was 100 and this number was already in residence, the successful life candidates had to await a vacancy. In the same year concern was expressed in the national press about the election system in general, though specific concerns were not raised about Earlswood. The unease related to fear about trafficking in votes, the methods used by professional canvassers and the administration of polling. However, the system continued to survive for many years.

Royal Patronage

The Royal Family supported the initiative to provide appropriate care for the learning disabled from the earliest days of the organisation. Prince Albert had already established a close relationship with Andrew Reed, lending his support to his earlier endeavours on behalf of the orphans of London.

Prince Albert visited Park House in March 1849. The Royal Consort was so impressed by the new initiative that he brought it to the attention of Queen Victoria who graciously agreed to meet members of the Society in 1850 to discuss their plans. As a result of the meeting Queen Victoria made a donation of 250 guineas to the Asylum, thus becoming entitled to name the occupant of one place in the Institution for the duration of her life. She accepted this in the name of her eldest son. The first recipient of her nomination was the son of a humble but exemplary minister amongst the Dissenters in Wales. A few months later she added a legacy of £500. When the Queen's donation was announced at the annual festival dinner in 1850 the levels of subscriptions increased dramatically.

In 1853 the Prince Consort laid the foundation stone for the main building at Earlswood. The Prince's only regret was the absence of the object of the Charity;

> **"whom, if it had been suitable, I should have liked to have welcomed here. But I will come again, and they shall see the Queen, when you are ready to receive us."**

In 1862 Queen Victoria granted Earlswood its Royal Charter, becoming Patron of the Institution.

Queen Victoria, Prince Albert and the Prince of Wales were not the only members of the Royal Family, aristocracy and nobility to lend their support to the charity. Support was provided in many ways. The Prince of Wales, H.R.H. the Duke of Cambridge, Lord Robert Grosvenor and Lord Carlisle were just a few of the influential Victorians who consented to preside at the annual festival dinners. Charles Dickens was persuaded by Dr. Conolly to accept the stewardship of one of the dinners at which funds were raised. Additional funds were gathered as a result of bazaars, these were organised and sponsored by the wives of the elite.

Queen Victoria's eldest son had laid the foundation stone for the first extension to the main building at Earlswood and her youngest son carried out the same duty for the final large extension of the century. The need for a detached infirmary had been recognised as early as 1866. However, it was not until the Committee had cleared the debt arising from the building of the 1869 extension that they felt able to begin this new project. In 1877 this had been achieved and plans were drawn up for the new building that was to be sited at the north-west corner of the existing buildings. The architects chosen were Lamb and Church of 12 South

The Asylum for Idiots,

EARLSWOOD, RED HILL, SURREY.

—◦•◦—

A BAZAAR

FOR THE SALE OF USEFUL AND ORNAMENTAL WORK,

To assist in the extinction of the Debt, will be held at the

HANOVER SQUARE ROOMS,

On SATURDAY the 2nd, MONDAY the 4th, and TUESDAY
the 5th of JULY, 1864.

Patronesses.

HER MOST GRACIOUS MAJESTY THE QUEEN.

HER ROYAL HIGHNESS THE DUCHESS OF CAMBRIDGE.
HER ROYAL HIGHNESS THE PRINCESS MARY OF CAMBRIDGE.

THE DUCHESS OF ST. ALBANS.	LADY CALTHORPE.
THE DUCHESS OF GRAFTON.	LADY CREMORNE.
THE DOWAGER MARCHIONESS OF SLIGO.	LADY PAUNCEFORT DUNCOMBE.
	LADY LOUISA FINCH.
THE COUNTESS OF ANTRIM.	LADY CHARLOTTE WENTWORTH FITZWILLIAM.
THE COUNTESS OF AYLESFORD.	
THE COUNTESS OF CALEDON.	LADY DOROTHY H. WENTWORTH FITZWILLIAM.
THE COUNTESS OF DARNLEY.	
THE COUNTESS OF ERROLL.	LADY CATHERINE HARCOURT.
THE COUNTESS OF HAREWOOD.	LADY LEGARD.
THE COUNTESS OF ILCHESTER.	LADY LOUISA MONCRIEFFE.
THE COUNTESS RUSSELL.	LADY C. MORANT.
THE COUNTESS OF SHAFTES-BURY.	LADY CAROLINE MURRAY.
	LADY MARIA PONSONBY.
THE DOWAGER COUNTESS SPENCER.	LADY GERTRUDE ROLLE.
	LADY MARY ROSS.
THE VISCOUNTESS COMBERMERE	LADY SANDYS.
THE VISCOUNTESS ENFIELD.	THE HON. MRS. R. F. BOYLE.
THE VISCOUNTESS JOCELYN.	THE HON. LYDIA F. C. DAWNAY.
THE VISCOUNTESS SYDNEY.	THE HON. MRS. D. PELHAM.
LADY BYRON.	

Treasurer.

MRS. RAINS, 21, King Edward's Road, Hackney.

Secretaries.

MRS. DOWNING, 61, Gracechurch Street, E.C.
MRS. EDWARD GRIFFITHS SYMS, Montpelier, South Lambeth.
MRS. LANGDON DOWN, Earlswood, Red Hill, Surrey.

Ladies' Committee.

MISS ARMFIELD.	MRS. LITTLE.	MRS. W. C. PRICE.
MRS. GAY.	MRS. MARTINY.	MRS. CHAS. REED.
MISS HOLLAND.	MISS MARTINY.	MRS. A. SAUNDERS.
MRS. C. W. C. HUTTON.	MISS MEAD.	MRS. SPENCE.
MISS JOLLY.	MISS ELEANOR MEAD.	MISS SMITH.
MRS. KELSEY.	MRS. PLUMBE.	MISS SYMS.
		MRS. WALKER.

Contributions of useful and ornamental work, clothing for the
poor, Irish knitting, paintings, prints, books, autographs, photographs, minerals, shells, feather, wax and paper flowers, wax fruit,
botanical specimens, turnery, stationery, cutlery, perfumery, glass,
china, fancy articles, and any light manufactured goods, will be
thankfully received up to June the 18th, and after that date at the
HANOVER-SQUARE ROOMS, to be addressed to the Secretaries of the
Bazaar for the Asylum for Idiots.

JOHN CONOLLY, M.D., D.C.L., *Hon. Secretary.*
WILLIAM NICHOLAS, *Secretary.*

OFFICE, 29, POULTRY, E.C.

Advertisement for bazaar

Place, Finsbury. The contract for the building work was signed with Messrs. Hall and Higgs of Crown Works, South Lambert.

The foundation stone was laid on the 11th of July 1877, the day of the Asylum's Annual Fete. Prince Leopold was accompanied by his equerry the Honourable A. Yorke, and his medical attendant Dr. Royle. The unfortunate Prince suffered from haemophilia and had never been strong. Born in the same year as his father laid the original foundation stone at Earlswood, he was to die in 1884, at only 31 years of age.

When the Prince arrived at Earlswood station the 5th Surrey Rifles, under Major King, provided a Guard of Honour. The Mayor and Corporation of Reigate were in attendance. Mr. Grece, the Town Clerk, read an address before the Prince entered an open carriage for the short journey to the Asylum. Mr. Abbiss, the oldest Board Member and first subscriber, was present for the service. For the short ceremony the Prince sat on the chair of the Grand Master of the Chief Lodge of Surrey, the chair previously used by his father and eldest brother. In a cavity beneath the stone the Prince placed a sealed bottle containing the last report of the institution, together with other documents and the coins of the realm. When the stone had been laid, Prince Leopold accepted as a gift the silver trowel that he had used in the ceremony. The Bishop of Guildford offered a prayer for the Royal Visitor and the Institution.

The guests partook of a luncheon in the dining room. Four toasts were made including one by the Prince himself for "the prosperity of the Institution and the Treasurer and Board of Management". He also mentioned the secretary Mr. Nicholas and Mr. Downing, the Collector. Following the luncheon the Royal party toured the hospital and visited wards, including those housing the three inmates maintained by the Queen.

The new infirmary was to have 42 beds in four large wards and three smaller rooms, together with a large day room. Sufficient donations of five pounds each had been contributed to provide 22 of the beds. The Bishop of Guildford, the Mayor of Reigate and Prince Leopold each donated one bed.

A bazaar was held in the main building with 22 stalls lining one side of the corridor. Goods to the value of £1,000 were offered for sale, the gift of the generous friends of the Asylum. Prince Leopold, before leaving the Asylum, toured the stalls and purchased three items. The bazaar remained open for three days.

Once the Prince had left the Institution the Annual Fete began. All of the usual attractions were present. Tea was served in the covered gymnasium and the day ended with a concert by the Earlswood Eccentric Exotics and Christy's Minstrels.

By April 1878 the new building was complete, requiring only the addition of the internal fittings. The final payment of £100 1s. 0d. (£100.05) was made to Lamb and Church on the 8th of August 1878. The Asylum received a receipt together with a note informing them of the death of Mr. Lamb on the same morning as the payment was made. Between August 1877 and August 1878 payments totalling £5,584 14s. 6d. (£5,584.73) were made to the builders, Higgs and Hill.

The Royal Family continued to maintain an interest in the Charity. In 1897 the double jubilees of Queen Victoria and the Earlswood Asylum were celebrated. Following the Queen's death in 1901 her son and daughter-in-law, King Edward VII and Queen Alexandra became Patrons of the Institution. Every monarch since has held this position, including our own Queen. When Earlswood was in desperate need of funds for a restoration programme in the first two decades of the twentieth century, King Edward VII graciously made a donation. In 1914 King George V, at the request of the officers of the Asylum, agreed that the name of the Institution should be changed from 'The Earlswood Asylum' to 'The Royal Earlswood Institution for Mental Defectives.'

Asylum Staff.

In 1853 the Asylum at Highgate employed 48 attendants and servants to care for 141 residents. Miss Ruddick was appointed to the post of Assistant School Mistress. She held the position for twelve and a half years before leaving, in February 1866, to get married. At the time it was still unacceptable for such a position to be held by a married woman. In recognition of her service she was presented with a leaving gift of twenty-five guineas in new gold and silver coins.

Early in 1856 the Commissioners in Lunacy strongly advised that the Asylum should draw up rules defining the duties of the officers and servants. A specimen of these is reproduced below. The staff had to adhere to very strict rules and the care of the residents was of utmost concern. No unreasonable force was to be used to control even the most difficult patient. Any officer seen striking a resident was immediately dismissed and, unless he was prepared to apologise, also rendered himself liable to prosecution.

Earlswood at the time housed 95 boys and 51 girls. The staff were listed as follows:

Schoolmaster	£100 with accommodation for self and wife but no board.
Steward/workshop	£80 with board and apartments in the house
Matron	£60 per annum.
Schoolmistress	£35 per annum.
Head attendant	£30 per annum.
4 attendants	£25 per annum.
2 attendants	£20 per annum.
1 attendant	£16.80 per annum.
1 houseman	£16 per annum.
Head nurse	£20 per annum
Second nurse	£18 per annum.
2 nurses @	£ 9 per annum.
2 nurses @	£ 8 per annum.
2 nurses @	£ 5 per annum.
1 nurse @	£ 4 per annum.
Head laundrywoman	£18 per annum.
Schoolroom maid	£ 7 per annum.
Kitchen maid	£ 8 per annum.
Wardrobe woman	£10 per annum.
Storeroom maid	£10 per annum.
Scullery maid	£ 5 per annum.
3 needlewomen	£12 per annum.
2 housemaids	£10 per annum.
1 housemaid	£ 6 per annum.
1 cook	£15 per annum.
5 women, 6 days @ 12.5 pence per day	
4 women, 4 days @ 12.5 pence per day	
12 labourers on farm–wages not stated	

Rules for Servants.

1. ALL servants will be engaged on probation for one month, during which period one week's notice will be sufficient. Those who have been permanently appointed, and whose services may be discontinued, will be entitled to one month's notice, or one month's pay; and they will be expected to give the same notice, or to forfeit one month's pay in the event of their leaving the service before the expiration of such notice.

Servants who may be suspended from duty are not entitled to any pay or rations during the period of suspension.

Servants are liable to be summarily dismissed for misconduct, without notice or claim.

2. All Servants to wear the livery of the Asylum during the hours of duty. The males to wear the jacket or coat buttoned throughout. The females to wear their caps in the manner prescribed by the matron. No crinoline to be worn. The hair to be plain and smooth.

The dress worn when out of livery to be neat and appropriate, and subject to the discretion of the Superintendent or Matron.

No Servant to go out of the building without a hat or bonnet.

Each person must send his or her clothes marked, to the laundry, accompanied by an inventory.

3. No communication is allowed between male and female Servants, except on the business of the Institution, during the hours of duty. No male Servant to go on the female side, and no female Servant to go on the male side without permission from the Superintendent or Matron.

The female Servants are to use the extreme west staircase only, and the outer door to the left of the dining-hall. The male Servants are to use the extreme east staircase only and the outer door to the right of the dining-hall. Standing or waiting at any time about the corridors, staircases, or entrance-doors is strictly prohibited.

4. The male Servants are not allowed to associate with the female Servants in the grounds. On alternate days male Servants, when off duty, will either remain in the building, or at once quit the Asylum premises.

On such days the female Servants will be permitted to take recreation in the grounds when off duty, but are to confine themselves to the paths or lower lawn. On other alternate days the female Servants will, when off duty at once quit the premises, or remain in the building; and on such days the male Attendants will be permitted to take recreation in the grounds when off duty. Servants are forbidden to enter the kitchen garden, farmyard, wilderness, or copse. Every Servant having obtained a permit must at once quit the premises.

5. The private Nurses and Attendants are not allowed to have any other Servant in their rooms at any time without permission. No Servant is to make a sitting-room of his or her bedroom, nor to have a fire there without the sanction of the Superintendent. No smoking is permitted before 8 o'clock p.m., and then only in the smoking-room.

6. No Servant is allowed to sing or whistle in the corridors or staircases. Bad language is strictly prohibited.

7. Generals Servants may read at breakfast and tea, but not at dinner. Nurses and Attendants taking their meals with patients are not permitted to read at those times.

8. No Servants, except those authorized, are allowed to do cooking of any kind.

9. No Servants are allowed to pluck plants, flowers, or fruit of any kind, whether wild or cultivated, without the sanction of the Superintendent, and they are required to restrict other, whether patients or servants, from destroying or mutilating the flowers, shrubs, or trees of the estate. Bird's nests are not to be interfered with.

10. Servants not rising at the proper time in the morning will have a portion deducted from their leave of absence.

11. No Servant is allowed to send a patient beyond the grounds without permission.

12. No Servant is allowed to employ patients to draw water, or empty slops, without special permission from the Superintendent or Matron.

13. Servants are not allowed to post letter or execute commissions for patients without permission. They are also forbidden to write or communicate in any way with the friends or relatives of an inmate.

14. No Servant is allowed to take charge of the money of patients, or to traffic with them in any way.

15. It is required that no Servant shall see or know of any patient being unkindly treated in any way, without reporting the same to the Superintendent.

Neglect or ill-treatment of a patient is a misdemeanour, and may be punished with imprisonment for a lengthened period.

16. The leave of absence granted to Servants is to be subject to the exigencies of the service of the Institution, and can never be demanded as a matter of right.

It is also liable to be partially or wholly withdrawn in the event of misconduct.

By Order of the Board

Resident Medical Superintendent

Staff regulations

With 17 nurses and attendants caring for 146 patients there was a ratio of patients to staff of just less than nine to one. In 1863 there were 350 residents with a ratio of two staff to every seven patients. The bill for salaries came to £3,000 per annum. In 1865 the Asylum had 120 male attendants, servants and officers and 130 female staff, mainly nurses, to care for the 420 residents.

In the early days the medical superintendent was not involved in the appointment of nurses or attendants. Dismissals were fairly common, particularly amongst attendants, and the main reason given was violence towards the children. However, there were other causes. In December 1849 an attendant was ordered to leave because he had arranged to marry the following day without seeking the approval of the Committee. In June 1850 an attendant and a house lad were accused of being out after the curfew hour. The house lad was dismissed. The attendant was only allowed to remain on probation, after he apologised, and he was demoted to a weekly servant. Drunkenness was also given as a cause for dismissal in some cases.

From January 1859 Dr. Langdon-Down supervised all of the appointments and the number of dismissals decreased significantly. In part this was due to changes made by Dr. Down who believed in the benefits of employing a small number of high quality staff. In 1869 the number of teachers employed within the school was reduced. However, the salaries paid to all attendants and servants were increased in order to ensure a better calibre of staff and to improve retention. By 1873 there was considerable difficulty in finding sufficient, quality staff, especially as better wages could still be earned elsewhere. The Commissioners in Lunacy recommended higher wages but it is uncertain whether an increase was made. Dr. Grabham, the Medical Superintendent, began to employ the wives of attendants to work on four of the boys' wards. The Commissioners in Lunacy noted a significant improvement in the care of the younger boys.

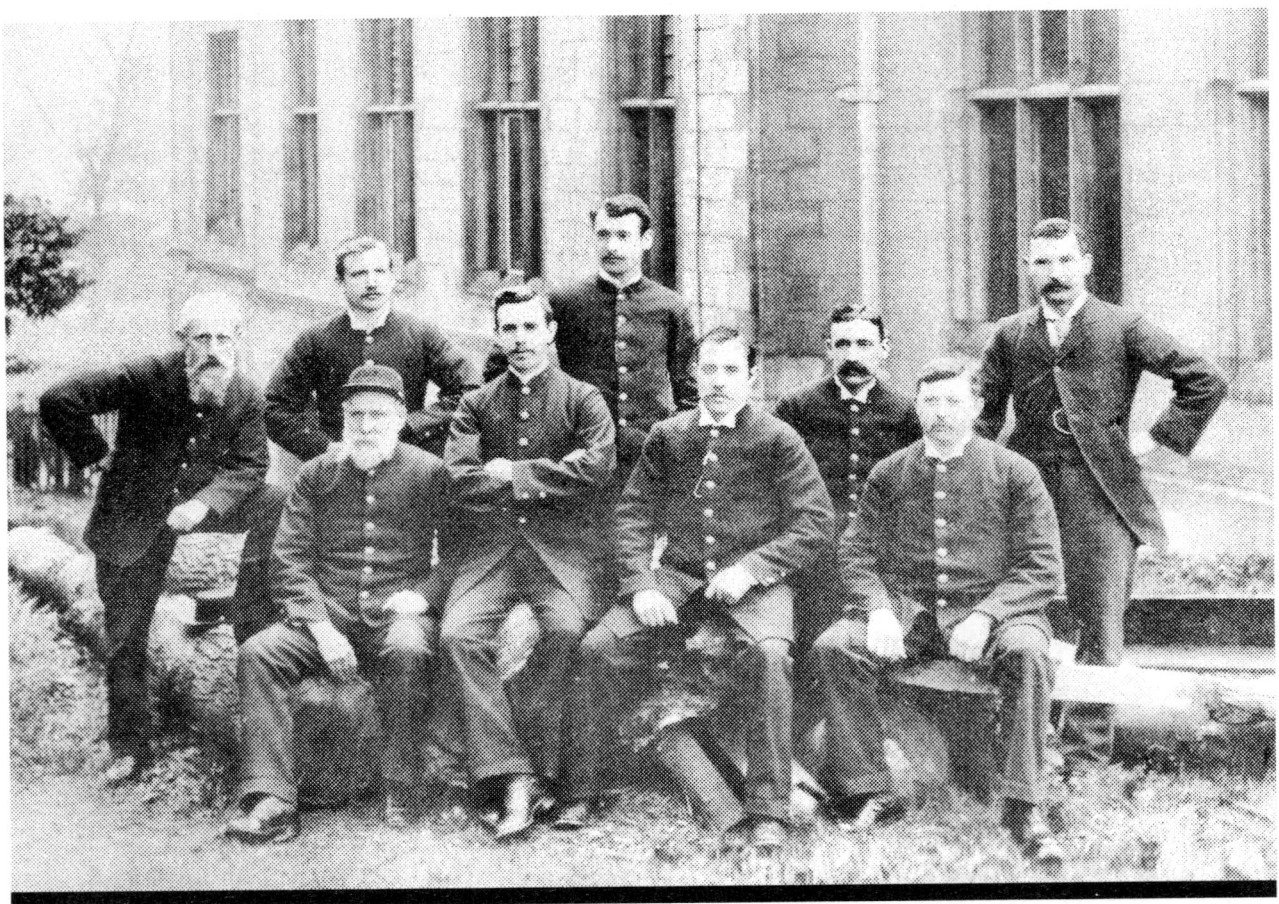

Attendants

Between 1868 and the 1881 a maid initially earned £10 per annum, a kitchen maid £12, a nurse £14 and attendants were employed at £25p.a. Salaries were increased by £1 per annum for up to five years. Only 15% of employees were born in Surrey. This was higher than average for domestic servants but lower than for staff at other hospitals. Forty-four percent of female staff stayed for six months or less. From 1874 Earlswood hired married couples, 22 in the first seven years. All other staff were unmarried.

Forty-three percent of male attendants were ex-service personnel, 12% had been attendants elsewhere, nine percent were labourers and two percent had been in service. Nineteen percent were artisans, employed at £30 per annum to work half time as attendants and the remainder in the workshops. Fifty percent stayed at Earlswood for less than 15 months.

In 1859 William Wood was appointed as Head Schoolmaster. He maintained a meticulous journal of everything that happened within the school. He kept records of the timetable and which teacher was to take each class. All outings were recorded including the names of the pupils who took part and the attendants that accompanied them. He worked out a detailed timetable and recorded all incidents that occurred. He even detailed the exact amounts of money that each child had available to spend on the outing and kept all of this information in his journal. From this source it is possible to gain a better understanding of how life was organised within the Asylum.

In addition to his work in the school he was closely involved with the Asylum band and choir. It was said to be much easier to obtain a position as an attendant in the Asylum if you were able to play a musical instrument. In his journal Wood recorded, for all attendants, any musical experience, instruments played, voice type and ability. He complained, in 1870, that the choir was so poor as a result of the fact that none of the male attendants could sing! In March 1878, after nineteen years at the Institution, he left to promote the 'Asylum for the Blind in Kent and Essex' at Gravesend. He was presented with a writing desk and a tea and coffee service that had been paid for by the staff and some of the more able residents. The committee's gift was a clock.

Mr. Brown was Steward of the Asylum and he had responsibility for the care of the estate and buildings. He had to keep daily records of the estate business and these were regularly presented to the management committee. It was the job of the Steward to "receive all provisions and other articles purchased or procured for the use of the Asylum, and before placing them in the store to examine and compare them with the bills of parcels or invoices severally relating thereto." He was also responsible for keeping the 'Admissions and Discharge Book' and the register in which was listed the religion or creed of every resident. He had to "superintend the various domestic departments, including the kitchen, and to take the general control of the labour of all the male patients who may be considered…to be fit for outdoor or domestic occupations." Duties also included, on the death of a patient, " to provide for the interment of the body." In the event of a violent death it was the Steward's responsibility to attend the coroner's inquest and report back to the Board. The Steward had overall responsibility for the behaviour, punctuality and dress of all the male staff, answerable only to the Medical Superintendent. He was also required to keep statistical and financial statements. The job carried with it immense responsibility and the workload must have been tremendous.

In April 1866, at the Annual Meeting at London Tavern, Mr. Brown was complimented on his overseeing the construction of the laundry extension and the new workshop building. It was a matter of great satisfaction that there had never been an accidental death at Earlswood.

To assist him in his work the Steward had a clerk and office boy. This person was required to work from 8.30a.m. - 6p.m. Monday to Saturday and "for such time on Sundays as may be necessary". He had six hours time off each week and 14 days leave per annum. During the six hours 'leave of absence' staff members were allowed to leave the Asylum. At all other times, despite being off duty, staff were required to remain on the premises. The leave of absence was allowed only at times acceptable to the running of the Asylum. Annual leave was not granted until 12 months service had been completed. The General Regulations stated that "Proposed marriages between servants or between servants and attendants must be notified to the Committee." Two employees who ignored this regulation were demoted. Staff could not receive visitors except in cases of illness or with the permission of the Medical Superintendent.

In 1870 Julia Goodwin was appointed as matron. She had, for the two previous years, been housekeeper at the Surrey County Lunatic Asylum at Brookwood. Forty-two percent of all female attendants and nurses had previously worked in hospitals or asylums.

The life was not easy for the staff at Earlswood. However, there were lighter moments. The Asylum provided for all aspects of life, both work and leisure, for both staff and residents. The staff enjoyed parties at the festive seasons. The following is a program for an entertainment that took place on the evening of the 25th of January, 1866.

In the early days of the Asylum the members of the Board were not only responsible for foundation of the Institution but also had direct involvement in the day-to day operation.

Alderman Abbiss was Treasurer, Mr. William Nicholas was Secretary, Andrew Reed, and later Dr. John Conolly, was the Honorary Secretary. They gave their time and their financial support unstintingly. The Commissioners in Lunacy were very supportive, thorough in their inspections and constructive in their advice. The non-resident medical officers also worked hard to make the Asylum an institution of which to be proud. Dr. Little, on a Saturday in June 1869, arrived at the Asylum late in the afternoon and stayed until most of the residents were in bed, his goal being to observe the workings of the establishment.

Servants Party
Supper at 8pm - sat down
Dancing commenced at 10.30pm
God save the Queen at 1am.
    1. Country dance
    2. Quadrille (1st set)
    3. Schottische
    4. La Farsoviana
    5. Lancers
        Games
    6. Waltz
    7. Polka
    8. Quadrille (2nd set)
    9. Schottische
    10. Sir Roger de Coverley

Program for evening entertainment

By the time of his last inspection report in 1889, Dr. Little was able to reflect on the progress that had been made at Earlswood from the "insanitary conditions and general unfittedness which it shared with most establishments in which large numbers of people were entertained day and night". It had exhibited "the atmosphere of a crowded lunatic asylum or workhouse of the time." He now was able to describe a place where "a stranger might, from the atmosphere of the interior, consider he was traversing a palace rather than the abode of a class of individuals incapable of helping themselves." He, however, recognised the need to continue the vigilance if standards were to be maintained.

By 1889 Earlswood was no longer the only institution of its kind in Britain. The Eastern Counties Asylum was established in 1859. The Starcross Asylum had been opened in 1864 in Exeter, and four years later the Northern Counties Asylum, known as the Royal Albert Asylum, had been founded in Lancaster. An early employee at Essex Hall, James Diggens, went on to have a long association with the latter. Earlswood was to be the model for all the new foundations that followed. The Royal Albert Asylum's first medical officer came from Earlswood and in 1885 the secretaries of the Eastern, Northern and Western Counties Asylums all visited Earlswood and ideas were exchanged.

Andrew Reed's death did not end the family's involvement with Earlswood. His son Sir Charles Reed took almost as much interest in the organisation as his father. He was born in Sonning, Berkshire and dedicated his life to the progress of education. Like is father he was very religious. Sir Charles became Chairman of the London School Board. His death occurred at 5.30am on the 25th of March in 1881 at his home, Earlsmead, in Tottenham.

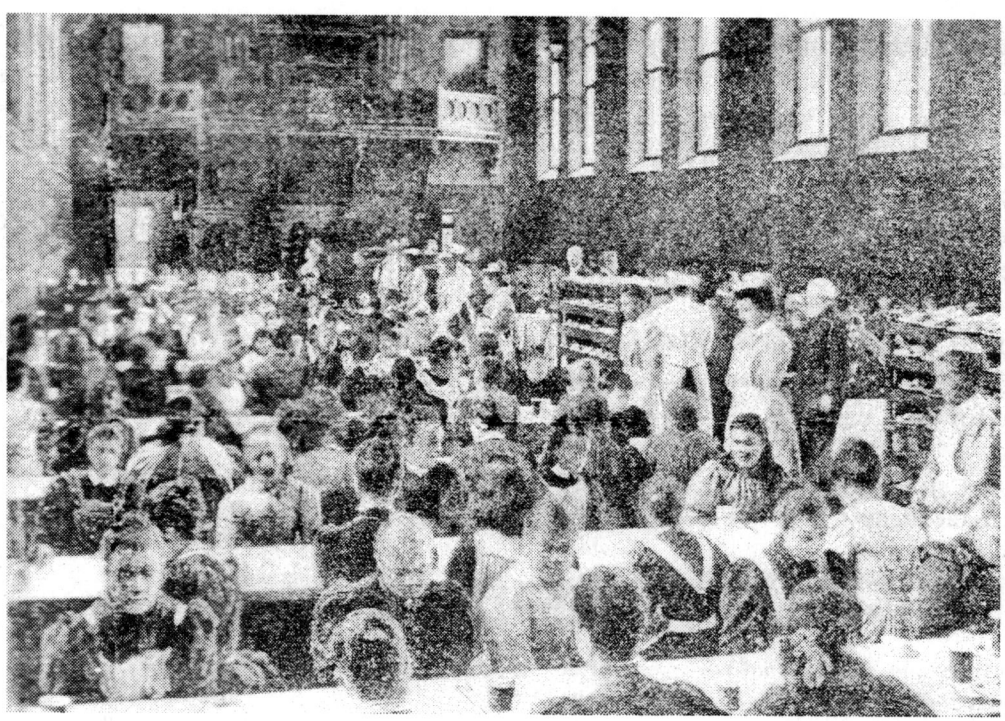

The dining hall

Shortly following the death of Charles Reed the Institution unfortunately lost another of its friends. James Abbiss had been born on the 3rd of June 1812 in Wallsworth, near Hitchin. He earned his living as a tea trader and became an alderman in 1859. In 1860 he was elected Sheriff of London and Middlesex. In addition to his support of Earlswood he also founded a Mechanics Institute. In early July 1882 Alderman Abbiss suffered a fit of paralysis and fell, hitting his head. He lingered for several days without recovering consciousness fully and he finally died on the 7th of July.

Mr. Small was head schoolmaster and religious instructor for 28years. Following his death in 1912, several newspapers carried details of his life. He had been born on the 26th of November 1820 in Cornwall. He was taken to London in 1824 by wagon, as the railway was still a thing of the future. He was originally refused employment at the London City Mission as he had heart disease. He was eventually appointed to the post when he undertook not to claim super-annuation in the event that he was taken ill. He continued in similar employment until he was appointed to Earlswood at the age of 63years in 1883. During his time at Earlswood Mr. Small was responsible for religious instruction and conducted Sunday Services and morning and evening prayers. As part of the traditional Annual Winter Festival in January 1911, Mr. Small's 90th birthday was celebrated and he was presented with a bound interlinear Bible and two other volumes, 'Scenes from the Life of our Lord' and 'The Gospel and the Old Testament'. Inside each volume there was an inscription that read;

> **"Earlswood Asylum. Presented to Mr. Thomas Small by the Board of Management, to commemorate his 90th birthday, and in appreciation of 28 years of zealous devotion as religious instructor to the patients and staff: New Year 1911."**

Mrs. Hull, the wife of the then Chairman of the Board, Mr. E.C.P. Hull, made the presentation. Mr. Small died on the 5th of January 1912, aged 91 years. A special grant of £100 was awarded to his widow in recognition of her husband's loyal service.

53

Harry Howard was appointed to the post of Secretary in 1875. He held the position for 50 years before his retirement. He died in 1942. Also employed in 1880 was Mr. Edis as house steward, Mr. G.T. A'vard as schoolmaster and Miss Hannah Parfitt as schoolmistress. The schoolmistress had responsibility for 123 small boys and 132 girls. Some of the older girls spent part of their time assisting the nurses in the dormitories, washing, dressing and feeding the helpless children, or with housework. They helped within the school, worked in the wardrobe or workrooms. They also helped to make the 555 beds every day.

In November 1891 the *'Earlswood Magazine'*, printed by the residents, recorded the marriage of Nurse Moyse and the Attendant Head and listed the members of staff who had over 20 years of service for the Charity.

Mr. Nice, (at Colchester)	over 38 years	entered	1 February, 1853
Miss Parker, (at Highgate)	" 36 "	"	19 February, 1855
Mrs. Nice, (at Highgate)	" 38 " (off and on)	"	1853
Mark Harper, }worked on first	" 36 "	"	June, 1855
W Comber, }buildings	about 36 to 37 years	"	1852, was away 2 or 3 years
Mr. David Harwood, (baker, cook)	over 33 "	"	May, 1858.
"Eliza Knight," (housemaid)	nearly 33 "	"	November, 1858
Mr. James Brinded, (Bricklayer)	over 32 "	"	1 October, 1859
Mr. James Smith, (sanitary inspector)	" 32 "	"	1859, at intervals before this.
Miss Dorcas Mann,	" 27 "	"	28 February, 1864
Miss Barlen, aged 73	" 27 "	"	21 June, 1864
Mr. Joseph Longhurst,	" 27 "	"	September, 1864
Mr. Alexander Edis,	" 25 "	"	6 September, 1866
Mr. William Smith,	" 25 "	continuously since 1870 & from 1860 to 1864	
Mr. Miller, aged 75,	" 23 "	since 1868	
Mr. James Mills,	" 23 "	entered June, 1868	
Miss Parfitt,	nearly 22 "	"	15 Nov., 1869
Mr. Henry Groves,	over 21 "	"	24 July, 1870
Mr. Henry Street,	" 21 "	"	20 August, 1870
Miss Caroline Habgood, (Nurse)	" 21 "	"	22 July, 1870
Mr. George Blundell, (Estate labourer)	" 21 "	"	24 July, 1870

In 1898 the staff regulations recorded the existence of a hall porter. His responsibilities included preventing any of the attendants, servants or other persons from loitering or gossiping in the entrance hall, ensuring that the doors were locked at all times, and preventing persons or property from leaving the building without the express permission of the Medical Superintendent.

A Day Gate Porter was employed to keep the gates and prevent the entrance or egress of any without authorisation, including dogs! His hours of duty were 6a.m. to 6p.m., unless there was no night porter, in which case he was expected to remain on duty until 10p.m. He had to record all comings and goings and inspect all parcels and goods, except those addressed to the principle officers. It was his responsibility to prevent staff from bringing any food in for the patients, and to exclude all alcohol from the Asylum. It was the duty of the Gate Porter to alert the Medical Superintendent or Matron to the late return of any staff absent on leave. Such a misdemeanour could result in dismissal for the staff member concerned.

Other staff employed included a coalman, a head and assistant seamstress, a cook who was responsible for ensuring the adequacy and quantity of food in the Asylum, firemen, a head laundress, laundry maids and mess room maids, responsible for all aspects of the food service to the staff. All appointments were the responsibility of the Committee and were probational for one month. When leaving the employ of the Asylum, staff were required, on the day of departure, to obtain a pass in order to be allowed to leave the premises. Many staff were accommodated within the Asylum and received lodgings and rations in addition to wages. If they chose, and were permitted, to live outside the Asylum a cash payment was made in place of the ration. The allowance for lodgings and washing were, in 1898, four shillings (20pence) per week. In the event of illness, staff received full pay for the first week and half pay thereafter, unless the Committee decided otherwise. Good conduct was rewarded by a bonus each quarter of ten shillings (50pence). Conversely, staff could be punished for misconduct by a reprimand, fine, suspension or dismissal. Drunkenness would always result in suspension, and if confirmed by the Committee, with dismissal. Some of the fines are listed below:

For coming late on duty or returning late from leave:-		
Not exceeding 10 minutes	6d	(2.5pence)
Not exceeding 20 minutes	1s 0d	(5pence)
Not exceeding 30 minutes	2s 6d	(12.5pence)
For not turning off light at proper time	Not exceeding 6d	(2.5pence)
For taking key off chain	Not exceeding 1s 0d	(5pence)
For neglecting to wear chain, with keys attached, while on duty	Not exceeding 5s	(25pence)
For losing a key	10s	(50pence)
For leaving a key on a hot water tap or anywhere in the bath room	10s	(50pence)
For allowing a patient to escape	The expense of recapture and any fine the Committee may impose.	
For losing regulations or being unable to produce them when called for	Such fine the Committee may impose.	

System of fines for staff

Uniforms were not issued to the staff until they had been employed for three months. They were inspected twice a year and replacements issued. The old uniforms then became the property of the staff except "in the case of male staff, the metal buttons are to be removed and handed to the Steward." The uniforms for the staff were made in the Asylums own workshops.

Income

The involvement of important public figures in the founding committee of the Charity ensured its early financial success. In spite of the outlay necessary for the acquisition of Park House, and the setting up of the establishment, funds allowed an investment of £822.50 in April 1848. Most of the money came from subscriptions and donations made at the first public meeting and first election. Funds continued to accrue, and by August 1853 at least £7000 had been invested in stock. The Charity's bankers were the Joint Stock Bank, Princes Road in the City.

For the first full year after the opening of Park House, expenditure totalled £4,424.38. Board and clothing accounted for £1,553.47, with £2,870.81 being spent on salaries, furniture, repairs, alterations, office rent, taxes, gas, washing, printing, advertisements, school books, stationery, postage and petty expenses. The receipts for the year amounted to £4,808.07, of which £3,441 was received from annual subscriptions and payments for pupils and £35.12 was collected when the Bishop of Oxford preached on behalf of the Charity.

Provision had to be made for the collection of subscriptions, donations and payments for pupils. In May 1848 Mr. Bedford was appointed as sub-secretary and collector. This proved to be an unfortunate appointment as the first auditor's report in February 1849 disclosed a deficiency of £72.15. He was immediately dismissed. Repayment of the money was requested but Mr. Bedford wrote to the Board detailing the 'distressing' nature of his situation. The Board sent him £5 "as an act of relief". Mr. Bedford's request for a testimonial was, however, refused. Shortly afterwards further irregularities were uncovered and the total debt was calculated at £120. Mr. Bedford had given two sureties when he was appointed. These were approached but failed to repay the debt. In the end the Charity was forced to take legal action against the first surety, Mr. Bedford's brother. He eventually repaid the money starting with a down payment of £20 in July 1850 and £10 per quarter for the following three years.

Following this, two separate individuals filled the posts of sub-secretary and collector. Their terms of employment, references and sureties were very carefully checked. Five percent of the subscriptions and donations were to be divided between them and they were guaranteed an income of £100 for the sub-secretary and £80 for the collector. The Board also decided on the wisdom of having a Finance Committee to deal with the Charity's financial affairs and regularly inspect its accounts. They decided that all maintenance payments should be made through the London Office, that receipts must be made out for all donations and subscriptions and that only an official receipt, signed by the sub-secretary, would be proof of payment of maintenance. Only the medical superintendent was permitted to have an account at the chemist and this was to be sent in quarterly and checked by him. The Charter decreed that three subscribers must audit the accounts.

For the first hundred years of the Charity all of the finance necessary for the construction and maintenance of buildings and the day-to-day running expenses had to be obtained in one of five ways; patient charges, subscriptions, donations, legacies and fund raising events. For example, in 1873 the total income for the year was £34,218 including £6,112 from subscriptions and £2,768 from donations. The Board and friends made special contributions, totalling £1,483.50, towards the development of new farm buildings. Legacies amounting to £5,883 were received, together with contributions of £1,007 to the building fund for the Infirmary. Life cases drew in £1,029 in maintenance. Gifts sometimes provided additional benefits that the Board were unable to provide. Amongst those received, from a wide variety of sources, were books, gardening tools, farm implements, a printing machine and even donkeys. Sir George and Lady Smyth generously treated all the inmates of Essex Hall to a "substantial dinner", whilst a Mr. Bunting gave them all a feast of strawberries. At Earlswood a Mr. Clarke funded the erection of farm buildings and initiated the farming of a section of the estate. The Society ordered a cultivator and the makers charged only half the usual amount. The London and Brighton Railway Company regularly provided carriage of goods and passengers at special rates.

In 1854 the New Philharmonic Society gave a performance in aid of the Charity and raised £50. However, the Board would not always accept the help offered. In 1857 an offer from a dramatic club to give a benefit performance was turned down, apparently the Board did not approve of the group.

Patient Charges

The amount of money raised from patient charges depended on the number of paying cases compared to those elected and accepted without payment. In 1862 pupil payments raised £6,994. The balance of cases accepted varied depending on the institution's need for funds. Initially, eligible cases could be guaranteed admission for the minimum sum of twenty-five guineas per annum. By the turn of the century the annual cost of a full payment place had risen to sixty-five guineas but a part-payment placement could be obtained for less provided a candidate could also attract sufficient votes.

	Payment cases £	Part Payment £	Life £	Misc £	Total Revenue* £
1862	6,994				21,657
1864					25,000
1865					30,557
1873			1,029		34,218
1874					31,221
1879					29,024
1883	8,507		1,913		30,120
1902	11,978	1,670		2,509	31,099
1903	12,206	1,788		4,122	31,581
1904	11,416	1,833		3,795	32,136
1905	10,841	1,770		2,228	31,664
1906	14,243	1,834		2,025	34,258
1907	12,274	1,742		2,101	34,020
1908	11,779	1,765		2,171	32,052
1909	11,811	1,932	750	2,224	26,594
1910	12,291	2,259		2,269	27,340
1911	12,940	2,555		2.035	27,915
1912	13,234	2,833	700	1,904	28,058
1913	13,409	2,813		2,260	35,532
1914	13,181	2,987		1,879	32,457
1915	14,571	2,991	1,116	2,108	26,883
1916	15,188	2,971		2,374	27,386
1917	18,170	2,921	1,056	3,522	35,603
1918	18,733	3,166		3,036	35,067
1919	22,807	3,545	630	2,965	38,230
1920	24,778	4,195		4,440	70,216
1921	25,827	4,653	1,000	4,318	60,327
					* includes legacies

Income from Patient charges

Between 1897 and 1901 the number of payment cases resident within the Asylum varied from 144 to 161, the average was 157. The income this generated ranged from £9,188 to £10,948, with an average income of £10,151 per annum. In 1902 concern over a shortfall in funding led to the suggestion of making a compulsory charge for every resident, even if it was only one shilling per week. There was provision from central sources for the care and protection of the 'afflicted poor'. Consequently, children from families in receipt of parish relief were ineligible for election. It was felt that Earlswood should concentrate on those whose families could contribute to their upkeep.

There were, in 1902, about forty vacancies on the female side. In a report the Medical Superintendent pointed out that £75 per case would generate £3,000 per annum. To fill these vacancies he advocated improved advertising. Large-scale adverts were not cost effective and direct mailing was favoured. In 1909 there were 267 residents who had been admitted without payment, 108 had paid up to 65 guineas, 25 had paid between 65 and 250 guineas, seven over 250 guineas and 34 were life payment cases. A funding crisis in 1910-11 resulted in the election of an unusually high number of part payment cases with a corresponding reduction in free places.

	Male	Female	Total
Life payment	8	13	21
Elected – payment	21	13	34
aided	114	52	166
Private payment			
Under £110	21	9	30
£110-£175	97	61	158
£175-£250	12	10	22
over £250	5	1	6
'Aided' payment			
Under £110	36	10	46
£110 & over	28	12	40
Grand total	342	181	523
Voluntary boarders			
Under £110	2		
£110-£175	3		5

Classification of Patients, 1938.

In October 1910 the Royal Commission estimated that there were 60,000 people with Learning Disability in Britain, 1000 of them in Surrey. It stressed the need for legislation to detain and supervise the 'feeble-minded' as it felt that families did not always understand the needs of the disabled. The General Court of the Charity expressed a willingness to admit 100 candidates at a special rate of one guinea per week if 'Council' and the education bodies recognised the benefit of such care. Many potential candidates were still confined within lunatic asylums. In 1939 *The Daily Telegraph* advertised "vacancies for those requiring Private Apartments and special attendants; also for Ordinary Private Patients at £110 p. a."

Subscriptions

Individual males	264	55%
Individual females	166	35%
Groups	4	1%
Anonymous	18	4%
Corporate	29	6%

Subscribers in the 1860s.

Annual subscription provided substantial funding. Numbers of subscribers always peaked after elections and festival dinners. Subscriptions trebled at the Festival dinner in 1850, following the announcement that Queen Victoria had pledged 250 guineas to the building of Earlswood. In the 1870s they reached an all time high, helping to offset reductions in income from other sources due to the Franco-Prussian war. Subscriptions increased from 5,000 in 1868 to 15,000 in 1876. Yet there was still a shortfall of £3,000 in income for 1875. The Prussian victory had a deleterious effect on the English economy. Bad harvests in the late 1870's and the trade depression in 1881 also impacted heavily on the Charity's income. Things had improved, however, by the end of the century. By 1900 the trustees had managed to invest funds sufficient to produce annual interest of £1,500. Much of the capital came from fees paid for life cases, which from 1873 onwards had been invested to cover the future expenses of these patients.

Seven percent of the subscribers were members of the gentry or aristocracy. The largest single subscriber was Samuel Morton Peto M.P. with 210 life votes.

	Annual	Life		Total
1873				£6,112
1879	£6,099	£4,416		
1883	£6,227	£4,624		
1897	£4,278	£1,303	- no fete	
1898	£4,357	£3,282		
1899	£4,324	£2,840		
1900	£4,401	£3,193	- no fete, special appeal	
1901	£4,416	£4,212		
1902	£4,398			
1903	£4,368			
1904	£4,131			
1905	£3,968			
1906	£3,824			£6,000
1907	£3,744			
1908	£3,708			
1909	£3,501			
1910	£3,474			
1911	£3,422			
1912	£3,346			
1913	£3,270			
1914	£3,147			
1915	£3,002			
1916	£2,843*			
1917	£2,553		* Contributions from elected cases	
1918	£2,605		stopped. Part payment only	
1919	£2,492			
1920	£2,174			
1921	£1,922			

Subscriptions.

Donations

Donations of any size were welcomed by the Charity and many were received without solicitation. However, on occasions the Board felt it appropriate to launch special appeals. One of the earliest was in 1854, for the building of Earlswood, when the following appeal was made:

> **"The Board have already received 270 patients and pupils, and they have upwards of 200 now knocking at their doors, and craving admission....the Board cannot look to complete this work of mercy with safety and prudence, except they can, during the erection, secure some £10,000 in addition to what they now have for the object."**

In April 1876 pledges of £3,425 for the Infirmary Fund were announced at the Annual General Meeting held at the London Tavern at which Alderman Abbiss presided.

Individuals and organisations of all sorts made donations of various sizes. In 1908 the Corporation of the City of London donated 200 guineas whilst the Royal Warrant Holders Association contributed £105. The following year the Poulters' Company gave 20 guineas and a further 10 guineas came from the Carpenters' Company. In 1910 a grateful patient sent a gift of £100 following his discharge. In 1918, for the third time, £100 was donated from the Queen Alexandra Day Fund on the instructions of the Queen

	Donations	Special Appeals	Total
1873	£2,768	£2,491	£5,259
1879	£1,532		
1880	£2,259		
1882	£2,631		
1883	£1,076		
1897	£ 690		
1898	£1,168		
1899	£1,464		
1900	£1,019		
1901	£1,391		
1902	£1,537	£2,427	£3,964
1903	£1,221	£2,936	£4,157
1904	£4,711	£4,321	£9,032
1905	£3,342	£4,500	£7,842
1906	£4,461	£4,134	£8,595
1907	£2,003	£2,924	£4,927
1908	£3,661	£1,696	£5,357
1909	£1,450	£3,160	£4,610
1910	£1,630	£1,715	£3,345
1911	£2,260	£2,150	£4,410
1912	£1,134	£2,441	£3,575
1913	£1,622	£2,073	£3,695
1914	£5,280	£2,237	£7,517
1915			£1,992
1916			£3,399
1917	£2,269	£3,190	£5,459
1918			£2,845
1919			£3,771
1920			£2,212
1921			£ 742

Income from donations.

Donations continued to be a significant source of income up to the closure of Earlswood. In 1969 donations received totalled £1066.75. Gifts ranging from £0.50 to £50 were received from individuals, whilst organisations as diverse as the Bishop Simpson School, the Clothworkers' Company, Bletchingley Womens' Institute, Horsham Methodist Wives Club and RAF Bands donated sums up to £80.

Legacies

Earlswood regularly benefited from legacies from its earliest days. Andrew Reed recorded:

"**Dec. 22. – Again I must gratefully acknowledge the good hand of God. A stranger... has just left us £2,000. He called at the office to see me during my**

absence, took away the Appeal and the Report of 1851, read them, altered his will in our favour, and died. Now may we move on."

In order to provide some security for the organisation a rule was applied that a quarter of the first £5,000 was invested, together with anything over that amount. The invested funds provided for capital expenditure that could not be met from normal income. The Board was required to hold a Special Court to obtain permission to utilise invested funds.

Income from legacies varied considerably year to year. Between 1897 and 1902 the income received from this source in any one year ranged from £1,700 to £17,000 with an average of £4,000 per annum. Approximately 20% of income came from legacies. Some legacies were left to the Charity with conditions applied. One such legacy founded the 'Servantes Trust'. Mrs. Anne Servantes left £2,500 in Trust to fund places for six children of Church of England clergy, barristers or solicitors. In 1910 this required the Trust to provide £90 per annum.

	Cash	Securities	Total
1861-2	£2,540	(£1,000 from Andrew Reed)	£3,540
1873-4	£5,883		
1879-80	£1,532		
1883-4	£1,076		
1901-2	£6,578		
1902-3	£4,938		
1903-4	£1,927		
1904-5	£5,013		
1905-6	£3,735		
1906-7	£9,230		
1907-8	£7,269		
1908-9	£1,764	* Ledgers prior to 1909 destroyed. No record of Securities	
1909-10	£3,700	transferred in payment of legacies.	
1910-11	£2,552		
1911-12	£2,465		
1912-13	£6,885	£3,198	£10,083
1913-14	£3,743		
1914-15	£ 668	£ 443	£ 1,111
1915-16	£ 610		
1916-17	£1,920		
1917-18	£4,432	£ 249	£ 4,681
1918-19	£2,018		
1919-20	£32,122	£ 382	£32,505
1920-21	£10,924	£10,940	£21,864

Legacies received.

In 1909 new legislation required ten percent of all legacies to be paid to the exchequer. This had a significant impact on legacies with income from this source falling by £3,000. Some legacies were very large indeed. In 1912 the *'Daily Telegraph'* reported that the hospital had debts of £4000 because of essential rebuilding work. In 1919-20 a William Henry Louis Ray bequeathed £60,000 to Earlswood. At a single stroke Royal Earlswood was clear of debt and a plaque within the hospital records this munificent act.

Fund raising events

Every opportunity was taken to raise funds for the Charity. At the laying of the first foundation stone in 1853 it was proposed that thirty gentlemen should lay 100 guineas each on the stone and two hundred ladies should each lay purses of five guineas or more on the stone, as part of the ceremony. Subscribers were also asked to double their subscription for five years, or make a special donation to aid the grand project.

A great supporter of Earlswood was the Reverend E Sidney, the Rector of Cornard Parva in Suffolk. He travelled around the country delivering his lecture on *'Earlswood and its Inmates'*. After hearing Sidney's address one man, who had planned to give five guineas, decided instead to give fifty. The Mayor of Liverpool donated 20 guineas. A total of £430 was raised in two days. A report of Sidney's lecture in the Liverpool Mercury on the 3rd of February 1863 quoted a poem, reputedly written by an inmate:

> **"Could we with ink the ocean fill**
> **Were the whole earth of parchment made**
> **Were every single stick a quill**
> **And every man a scribe by trade**
>
> **To write the love of God above**
> **Would drain the ocean dry**
> **Nor could the scroll contain the whole,**
> **If stretched from sky to sky."**

By 1863, helped by donations collected during these lectures, the building debt had been reduced from £20,000 to £9,000 and it was hoped to clear the debt within a year. The Members of the Board themselves pledged £1,500. *(The debt was indeed cleared by early 1865.)*

The scale of the operation is impressive. In 1865, when Sidney was to deliver his lecture in Bristol, 1500 circulars were produced together with 1000 of the pamphlets that would be handed out at the meeting. 500 bills were given to shops and 250 posters distributed. A leaflet and letter was sent to 150 clergymen asking them to announce the lecture. The meeting generated £350 of income.

It could be said that Earlswood invented 'the Road Show'. In order to attract more funding, by enlisting additional subscribers, a team toured the industrial towns of the North holding public meetings in each town. Presentations were held describing the work and the achievements of the Institution. Examples of the articles produced by the inmates were on show for the audience to inspect and purchase. In 1862 over £150 was raised by a sale of work produced by residents.

The Guilds and trade organisations were encouraged to subscribe. Fifty pounds per annum was sufficient to ensure that, if a member's child should require admission and was a suitable candidate, a place could be guaranteed. Trades and merchants were exhorted to give money so that a town could elect a child each year. In November 1862 just such a public meeting was held in Bradford. The Chairman W.E. Forster Esq. advocated the setting up of an Asylum in the north to parallel Earlswood, as it was obvious that one institution could not serve the whole of the country. However, in the interim he advocated that support be given to Earlswood. In future years the Royal Albert Asylum was established on the same lines as Earlswood.

The following day a meeting was held in Sheffield and *'The Sheffield and Rotherham Independent'* reported that inmates gave a demonstration of drill that was a match for any militia or rifle company. The Duke of Wellington viewed just such an exhibition and it was reported that he was 'impressed'. The following day Huddersfield was the venue for the next in the gruelling series of fund raising meetings. Earlswood drew support from all over the country. In 1862 Yorkshire sent more money than any county except Middlesex. In November

1863 Newcastle set up its own committee to raise funds. The town had three children within Earlswood.

Efforts were underway in all parts of the country. In 1866 the 'Road Show' visited Oxford. The Bishop of Oxford presided and £188 was raised in the collection. In 1867 a Public Meeting was held in Brighton. In March 1875, at Ryde on the Isle of Wight, Mr. W Nichols gave a lecture on the daily life of the institution to raise funds for the re-election for life of John Elliot Long. A further Public meeting was held that year in Torquay. In July 1876 a Public Meeting was held in Eastbourne and a further one in November in Brighton. In 1877 a meeting in Canterbury was presided over by the Dean of the Cathedral. The Mayor and many other important men of the town attended. In 1882 a public meeting was held at Market Harborough. In 1883 one was held in Cardiff and the Bishop of Llandaff gave the address.

On the 2nd of April 1864 the *West Surrey Times* carried a notice announcing that Earlswood planned to hold a Bazaar on the 2nd, 4th and 5th of July under the patronage of the Queen, the Duchess of Cambridge and Princess Mary of Cambridge. Contributions were requested. The admission to the Bazaar was one shilling (five pence). There were various stalls. The Prince and Princess of Wales attended at midday and stayed for an hour. The event was then opened to the public. It was at this event that Alderman Abbiss first informed the Prince of the plan to extend the building the following year and the Prince agreed to return and lay the foundation stone. On the 11th and 12th of November 1864 a further Bazaar was held in the Guildhall with the same patrons as that in July. The Mayor and Mayoress of London visited on the first day. There were 27 stalls, one under the supervision of Mrs. Plumbe, so important in the original foundation; Mrs. Down, wife of the Medical Superintendent, Dr. Langdon Down, managed a second.

On the 7th and 8th of April 1875 a bazaar was held in the Town Hall at Banbury. Goods produced by the residents of the Institution were offered for sale on a number of the stalls. Refreshments were provided by the townspeople. The events raised £290 for the Asylum. In June 1879 an auction of china and bric-a-brac took place in Nottingham over a period of three days. The proceeds were divided between Earlswood Hospital and a Lincolnshire charity. The donations to the sale included some rare Oriental and European china.

Another kind of fund raising event was the Festival Dinner. These were held annually in spring and were prestigious events, attended by many people from the top ranks of society. The Charity seemed to have no difficulty engaging well-known and important celebrities to preside. In 1871 the Prince of Wales agreed to take this role. In 1851 Charles Dickens had consented to become one of the Stewards at the dinner. Money was raised both by the sale of tickets and by subscriptions. The dinner in 1863 saw subscriptions of £2,000, whilst that on the 28th of February 1866 produced £2,300. The next year saw record subscriptions. Initially, the 200 people attending the dinner pledged £4,900. The Lord Mayor of London, who was presiding, offered to give a further five pounds if nineteen other people would do the same. The challenge was accepted and £5,000 was declared for the evening.

In 1877 £3,613 was raised including £50 from the Director and staff of the Bank of England. In 1878 the Festival Dinner was held at the Albion Tavern in Aldersgate Street. One hundred and twenty people attended and £1,594 were raised. The following year the dinner was held at the same tavern, Baron Henry de Worms was in the chair; £2,900 was raised including £500 in a single anonymous donation. In 1880 the festival raised £2,259. In 1883 the 36th Anniversary festival dinner was once again held at The Albion in London. The infirmary, designed to hold

63

fifty beds, was still unfurnished due to lack of funds. The 120 people who attended pledged a total of £1,000. In 1908 nearly £2,000 was given on the night. The following year £3,100 was pledged in subscriptions. In 1910 and 1911 subscriptions of £1,692 and £2,110 respectively were announced. In 1969, the Mayor of Reigate and Banstead hosted a charity ball. More than 600 guests attended and raised £1,100.

In 1923 the Board of Management was forced to look closely at income and expenditure as costs were rising. The income that could be relied upon was made up as follows:

Payment cases	£26,000
Part-payment cases	£ 4,600
Miscellaneous receipts	£ 4,000
Subscriptions and donations	£ 1,400
Dinner	£ 3,000
Total	£39,000

The charges for payment cases ranged from £110 to £375 per annum. Those eligible but unable to pay these charges could be admitted for 25 or 60 guineas depending on circumstances. Free election cases had been abolished due to new legislation. For this and other reasons the income from charitable contributions had been considerably reduced. A revision of payment charges was recommended.

Other Income.

Shoe	£132.25
Tailor	£83.63
Print	£55.20
Basket	£2.95
Brush	£4.78
Mat/mattress	£3.14
Total	£281.95

Profit from the workshops within Earlswood in 1883

Contributing to the income generated by the Institution was the profit earned by the various workshops within the institution. Earlswood also generated small amounts of money by leasing property that it held, but for which it had no other use. In 1872 the Asylum leased a cottage on Earlswood common for £30 per year to a William Church. In 1874, the Asylum sublet the back room of 36 King William Street, its London headquarters, to David Bumsted and John Campbell Bumsted for use as an office, at a rent of £70 per annum.

By 1950 the list of properties being let, included:

Princes Road houses	Superintendent's Quarters, Farmfield
Back Lodge, Princes Road	4 Ireland Cottages, Redhill
Farmfield Cottages	Farm House, Royal Earlswood
Kiln Cottage, Farmfield	Farmfield Lodge
Brook Cottage, Lonesome Lane	Flats, Lonesome Lodge, Lonesome Lane
Lonesome Farm, Lonesome Lane	

In 1913 the Mental Deficiency Bill was passed requiring provision to be made for the mentally handicapped. Central government provided £150,000 per annum, sufficient for 20,000 cases.

Local authorities were expected to provide an equal sum. This put a halfpenny in the pound on the rates.

Expenditure.

As well as income, great care had to be taken to control expenditure. Funds were always limited and the Board was determined to optimise their purchasing power. All stores were centrally organised, for food, clothing, linen, boots etc. Classes or wards carried no stock of their own, receiving daily issues as appropriate. This allowed for very close control with minimal wastage and was generally very successful. In 1864 the income raised was £25,000, the expenditure £21,500.

Year	No of Inmates	Average cost per head Housekeeping	Total cost per head	Total annual expenditure.
1850	117	£29.54	£60.94	£ 7,129.93
1857	274	£23.59	£42.84	£11,738.03
1867	438	£29.13	£46.18	£20,225.56
1877	609	£23.77	£47.68	£29.037.50
1887	569	£21.36	£47.63	£27,103.38
1897	572	£22.48	£49.28	£28,191.67

Examples of costs and expenditure

In 1879 receipts totalled £29,024, including subscriptions of £6,099, life payments of £4,416, donations totalling £1,532, legacies of £3,526 and £9,481 from the pupils' account. Meanwhile expenditure on housekeeping, clothes, medicine and laundry was controlled at £15,725, wages for schoolmasters and servants amounted to £2,927, whilst wages for other staff, commissions and office expenditure cost £1,514. A year of good receipts halved the Asylum's outstanding debt from £5,000 to £2,500.

Financially 1883 was to prove another successful year.

Annual subscriptions	£6,227	Housekeeping	£14,779
Life subscriptions	£4,624	Wages	£2,891
Donations	£1,076	Salaries	£1,479
Legacies	£4,562	Wear and tear	
Charges for board of pupils	£8,507	of furniture	
Charges for maintenance		& miscellaneous	£1,337
of life cases	£1,913		
Miscellaneous	£3,211		
Total receipts	£30,120	Total expenditure	£27,836

Receipts and expenditure in 1883

Things did not always go so well. In 1902 there was concern over the institution's expenditure. A special resolution was passed on March 12th requiring

> **"That our Medical Superintendent and our Secretary be requested to make a thorough investigation of the system of expenditure and financial management of the entire institution, with full powers, and to make a report thereon to the Board in due course."**

The report that was produced later that year was impressive in its attention to detail. It recommended that the day-to-day running of the institution be in the hands of the Medical Superintendent, and that he should have two Assistant Medical Officers to permit him the time to manage other affairs. The Medical Superintendent would supervise all the meat ordering. Discrepancies over the previous years indicated that this would provide savings of approximately £1,000 per year. Beer consumption had varied from 4,117 to 6,178 pints per annum. The laundry had washed 11,500 articles in one year and 13,000 in the next, yet 227kgs (500lbs) of soap and 164kgs (360lbs) of soda had been used in both years. The Asylum had used 97tons of potatoes in 1900 and 83tons in 1901. The report detailed the following:

Potatoes if scraped lose	4%
if machined lose	16%
if peeled lose	25%

By scraping or machining it had been determined that 70tons of potatoes would be adequate.

Year	Cost	Year	Cost
1849	£36.39	1869	£20.88
1850	£29.54	1870	£21.41
1851	£22.71	1871	£23.63
1852	£21.38	1872	£23.47
1853	£22.66	1873	£23.41
1854	£22.60	1874	£22.03
1855	£19.93	1875	£21.19
1856	£25.77	1876	£23.41
1857	£23.59	1877	£23.77
1858	£21.97	1878	£23.66
1859	£21.60	1879	£24.27
1860	£22.32	1880	£23.31
1861	£26.25	1881	£23.64
1862	£26.88	1882	£23.87
1863	£26.21	1883	£24.23
1864	£26.70	1884	£22.26
1865	£27.39	1885	£20.95
1866	£28.42	1886	£22.35
1867	£29.13	1887	£21.36
1868	£27.71	1888	£21.11

Annual Housekeeping Costs per Head 1849-1888.

It was noted that gas was supplied free to staff, leading to wastage. Metering was recommended. Coal was used to provide light and heating for the building. Consumption had been reduced from seven and a half to six tons per day as a result of supervision. The farm bailiff supplied food to the institution and charged what he liked. Dorchester Asylum farm provided 3,884kgs (8,540lbs) of meat per year at the equivalent of four and a half pence (2p) per kilogram. Earlswood could not compete with this. The Royal Albert Asylum produced milk at just over three pence (1_ p) per gallon, the price at Colchester Asylum was less than four pence (1_ p) per gallon, whilst Earlswood farm charged five pence (2p) per gallon. In addition the amount supplied ranged from 70 to 82 gallons per day whilst the requirement for the number of inmates resident at any time was estimated at 60-66 gallons daily.

Per capita housekeeping costs fell as the number of residents increased. Spending on different household items, as a proportion of the whole cost, varied considerably over the years.

Item	1849 (£)	1868 (£)	1888 (£)
Bread/Flour	3.25	3.18	1.51
Meat	6.73	6.26	7.77
Butter/cheese	1.95	1.41	1.05
Groceries, soap etc.	2.67	1.42	1.31
Milk	1.48	1.77	1.55
Potatoes	1.52	1.28	0.93
Beer/wine	2.10	0.98	0.93
Coals	0.94	3.45	2.16
Clothing	8.05	5.51	-
Washing	4.66	1.48	2.28
Drugs/chemicals	0.54	0.20	0.15
Gas	0.46	0.48	1.03
Water	1.55	0.23	0.08
Sundries	0.83	0.13	0.37
Total Housekeeping	36.39	27.71	21.11

Composition of Costing.

By 1910 the Institution needed an annual income of £28,000. Forty pounds per day was required from voluntary subscription to support those of the 500 inmates who were wholly or partly dependent on charity. 1915 saw a further crisis in funding, due to the war, with costs increasing by 15% and subscriptions falling. Income fell to less than £27,000. The Institution found it necessary to raise £15,000 in loans. The averaged annual figures indicate the effect of the war on income and expenditure. Income did increase again in 1917 and a large bequest in 1919/20 enabled the Institution to discharge its debts. In 1926 total receipts were £52,312 11s (£52,312.55) and total expenditure was £52,019 18s 8d (£52,019.93).

1889-92	Receipts	
	Expenditure	£28,072
1902-6	Receipts	£32,147
	Expenditure	£27,793
1907-11	Receipts	£29,584
	Expenditure	£28,179
1912-16	Receipts	£30,063
	Expenditure	£30,370
1917-21	Receipts	£47,888(i)
	Expenditure	£40,647

Averaged annual income/expenditure.

Costs remained high after the war years. Expenditure in the Royal Earlswood Group outstripped that of other similar hospitals, in 1955 the cost per head per week at Earlswood was £5 10s (£5.50) compared with an average for the region of £4 18s 1d (£4.90) and for England & Wales £4 12s 1d (£4.60). By 1968-9 the gross expenditure for the Royal Earlswood Group, excluding capital items, was £894,115.

(i) including large bequest in 1919/20

Item	£
Housekeeping	20,000
Advertising	550
Clothing	4,300
Annual Festival	300
Salaries, Institution	3,660
Wages do	6,570
Salaries, Office	1,270
Travelling expenses and carriage	150
Insurance	235
Rates and Taxes	1,470
Pensions	845
Upkeep of grounds	250
Office rent	220
Printing and stationery	400
Postage and sundries	150
General repairs. Buildings	1,800
Plant and machinery	530
Furniture – replacements etc.	
Institution	1,500
Office	10
Total	£44,210

Expenditure in 1922.

Item	£
Salaries and wages	560,073
Provisions	82,644
Uniforms and clothing	23,612
Drugs, dressings etc.	8,954
Fuel, Light, Power, Water and Laundry	57,338
Maintenance of building, plant and grounds	73,254
Domestic repairs, renewals and replacements	21,097
Other Expenses	894,115

Expenditure for year ending 1969

The cost per head increased rapidly over the following years, affected by inflation:

1966-67	£13 4s 4d (£13.22)
1968	£14 2s 5d (£14.12)
1969	£15 9s 3d (£15.46)
1970/1	£17 9s 3d (£17.46)
1971/2	£22 0s 7d (£17.03)
1973	£26 3s 5d (£26.17)
1974	£28 11s 0d (£28.55)
1975	£32 16s 5d (£32.82)

Expenditure per head, per week from 1966-1975

PROFIT AND LOSS			
Drawn.			
Dec 31.1864			
To Housekeeping Expenses for Board, Clothing,	£	s	d
Coals, Washing, Medicine &c.			
	9,406	5	7
Salaries of Officers, Earlswood and Office,			
Commission, and all Office Expenses			
	2,150	15	9
Wages – Attendants, Masters of Trades and Servants	949	15	7
Furniture, including Bedding, Linen, Earthenware,			
Hardware, fittings &c			
	913	16	4
Repairs, Painting, Colouring, Varnish &c	345	11	8
Printing Lists of Subscribers, Reports, Proxies,			
'Visits to Earlswood', Lectures &c			
	286	18	11
Stationery, Office and Asylum, School Books &c	155	5	6
Advertisements	331	17	5
Postage of Proxies, Reports, Circulars, Letter &c.	200	0	0
Carriage of Goods, Materials and Travelling Expenses	207	3	4
Rates and Taxes	225	16	3
Legal Expenses (Legacy)	127	6	8
Gas	172	4	2
Insurance	17	6	0
Expenses of Public Meeting, Birmingham	76	4	1
Interest on Loans	315	8	5
Workshops' Expenses	48	6	4
Rent, Office	60	0	0
Funeral Expenses	75	8	8
Furniture, Office	18	8	6
Estate, Repairs to Roads, Paths &c.	150	0	0
Miscellaneous Expenditure	166	8	10
Balance to Capital	14,157	3	6
	30,557	11	6
Credit			
Dec 31. 1864	£	s	d
By Pupils account, Charge for the Year	7,815	5	6
Annual Subscriptions	4,672	6	1
Life	2,019	2	6
Donations	1,184	6	7
Miscellaneous Receipts	536	1	0
Legacies	4,054	5	6
Life Payment Cases	520	0	0
Gift from Debt Fund	9,307	0	0
Kitchen Garden	40	15	4
Farm	408	9	0
	30,557	11	6

BALANCE SHEET				
Drawn	Assets	£	s	d
Dec 31. 1864				
To Pupils' Account, Amount due		1,032	17	6
S.E. Railway Stock		450	0	0
Metropolitan Association Shares		125	0	0
Banker's Account		1,350	3	3
Petty Cash Office		1	5	11
Deposit Account		2,000	0	0
Steward		51	17	1
Workshop, Stock in Hand &c.		219	11	0
Building		57,899	5	0
Estate		12,653	9	10
Plant and Machinery		2,159	4	5
Furniture, Office		129	0	0
" Earlswood		6,396	14	9
Timber in Stock		80	12	11
		84,549	1	8
Credit	Liabilities	£	s	d
Dec 31. 1864				
By Life Payments received		4,642	10	0
Christmas Bills due		3,377	3	2
Capital Account		76,529	8	6
		84,549	1	8

Example of Balance Sheet for Earlswood Asylum

Education

Education was an important goal of the Institution. The lessons were to be very practical and were designed to improve life skills and health. The children were encouraged to exercise and the formal lessons included the three R's, language and shop keeping. The children had a counter and acted as buyers and sellers. In this way they learned about supplies, money, numbers, weights and measures. The Commissioners of Lunacy suggested the teaching of geography by using "a good plan of the grounds, and several portions of the establishment or neighbouring district with which the pupils are familiar." The annual report in 1853 reported that:

> **Ninety-eight are daily engaged in reading and spelling.**
> **Eighty-six in writing.**
> **Twenty-five in drawing.**
> **Twenty in gardening.**
> **Twenty-eight in sewing, knitting etc.**
> **Sixteen boys in willow-plaiting.**
> **Five boys in each class are respectively basket-makers,**
>   **shoemakers and tailors.**
> **Six are daily occupied as carpenters.**
> **Sixteen are engaged in domestic work.**
> **Twenty take lessons in dancing.**
> **Seventy have object-lessons.**
> **Eighteen write from dictation, and learn geography and arithmetic.**
> **A hundred and one are drilled, and take gymnastic exercises.**
> **Thirty-nine have speaking lessons.**
> **A hundred and forty-nine attend domestic worship.**
> **A hundred and four attend public worship.**
>
> **The greater part of the family are practised in singing, and some are taught on the harmonium.**

The discipline was described in the *'Daily Telegraph'* on the 20th of August 1862 as "military but motherly". They reported that the children were "Drilled in behaviour, lessons, routine and work".

In 1864 the *London Mirror* described the girls lessons as follows:

> **"Additional means of instruction have been introduced into the girls' school. Efforts have been successfully used to make the teaching of domestic work a part of the school lessons. Bedmaking, scrubbing and processes of daily life are systematically taught and afford agreeable diversion from the more strictly scholastic work."**

Girls were not the only ones to learn household skills, fourteen boys also received instruction in housework. Forty-six girls were taught needlework, made bead mats and other fancy articles.

The younger children attended school full time whilst the older ones had school for half a day and worked in one of the institution workshops for the other half. In 1866 there were 102 in the girls school. The schoolmaster's report in November of that year listed 141 in the boys' school, 20 full time and 121 half time (one week in the morning and the next in the afternoon). Seventeen could read well and 29 could read slowly. Eighteen can write sentences and 35 copy simple words. Eight could calculate sums, whilst 20 could do addition and count above 100. Sixty-five were familiar with coins and knew some weights and 26 could tell the time at least to the hour.

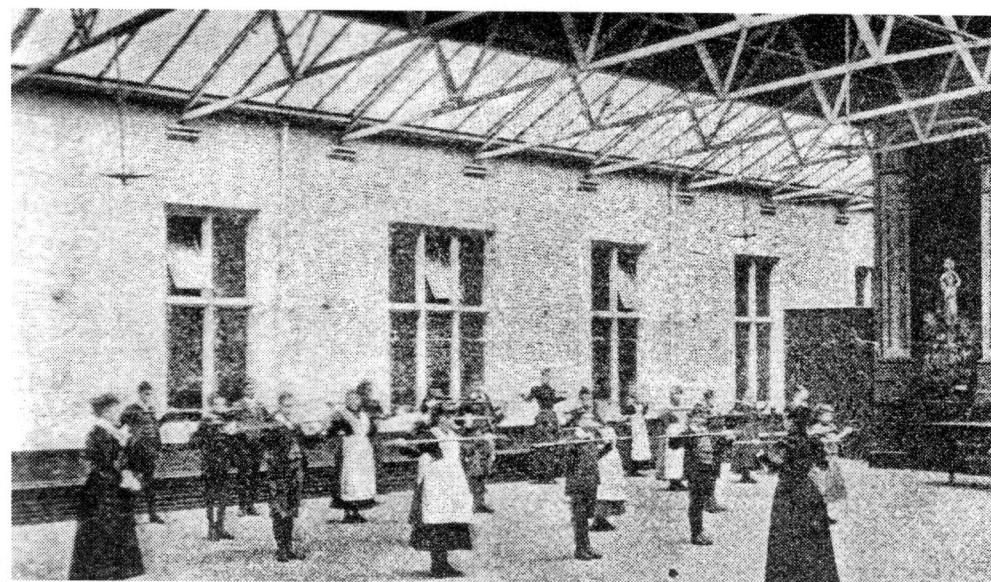

The exercise yard

In 1872 lessons were being given on speaking, reading, writing, arithmetic, drawing and music. Many of the children had to be taught their own name, how to dress themselves and other daily routines. In 1879-80 there were five classes. The girls' timetable included 25 minutes practising speech, 75 minutes of mental work, 78 minutes of industrial and handicraft work, 30 minutes of physical education, 20 minutes of music, dancing and singing and eight minutes of recreation in every four hours of classes. To encourage literacy and an interest in the outside world the Asylum subscribed to a number of periodicals and provided a reading room.

By 1883 there were 123 young boys and 132 girls under the care of the schoolmistress. There were 111 boys in the continuation school, 51 full time, 57 half time and 3 occasionally. The schoolmaster recorded that 92 were able to drill and march, 34 could read and write well and 19 could read a little. Lessons were 35 to 45 minutes long, three in the morning and three in the afternoon. In between lessons the children gathered together for singing, exercises, movement and music and information on money and multiplication tables. Those who could read had the Bible and lesson books, the lower classes read from a board collectively. In 'shopkeeping' they studied weighing, pricing and selling. Pupils were examined every six months.

The boys' continuation school was responsible for managing the letters and cards arriving at and leaving the hospital. In 1883, 508 letters left the hospital, 255 were written by the residents themselves and 253 by others on their behalf.

'The Quiver' in 1899 reported that:

> **"...the Head Governess is of the opinion that the little ones are never happier than when they are at lessons. According to their ability, they go through the course usually adopted in elementary schools, and have the same physical exercises. The elder girls are employed in housework or in the laundry. Many, no doubt, enjoy the new experience of being usefully employed, and industry and willingness are rewarded by an afternoon walk to the town, a small amount of pocket-money, and a reward at the New Year."**

At Earlswood education was viewed as essential. In 1911 there were about 150 children in the junior and main school. In 1913 the Mental Deficiency Bill made the education of learning disabled children compulsory everywhere. Local education committees were given the task of providing care and an education appropriate for the individual child.

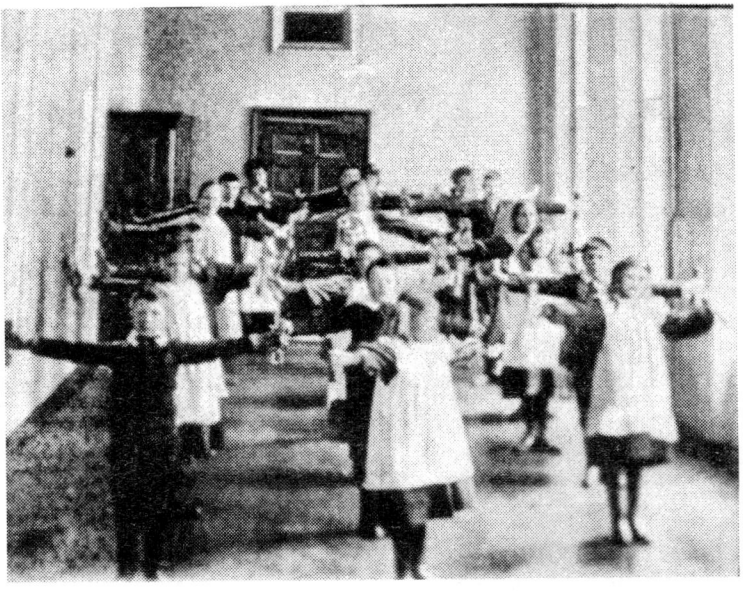

Drill class

The school only took those who were considered to be educable and children had to be seven or eight to attend. One of the teachers, a Miss Brooker, had the idea to incorporate the infants. The nursery was started in a tin hut, the annexe, in 1923-4. When Bridge House became vacant following the completion of the term of a private letting, Mrs. Yearsley, the Head Teacher, requested its use for the senior school. The nursery, which was composed of six classes, moved into the vacated school accommodation in the main building. Miss Brooker was later to leave to start the school at St. Lawrence's in Caterham. Mrs. Wells, prior to her marriage, ran the nursery, helped by nurses. When she left to get married, the infant and intermediate classes moved into Bridge House under Mrs. Cunningham.

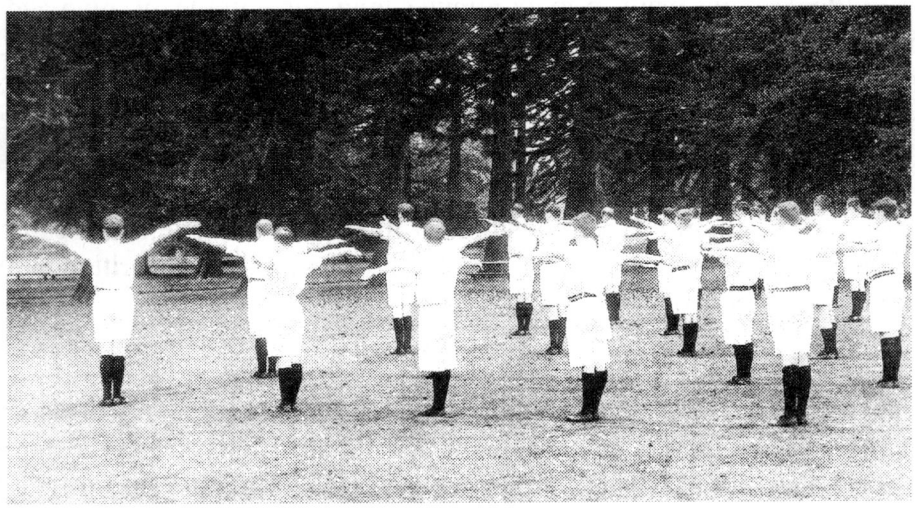

An exercise class

For the older girls, the emphasis was on teaching handicrafts that would provide a means of earning a living. Staff taught machining and embroidery and the matron gave lessons in Honiton lace making. When Earlswood Home at Walton closed during the war, its matron came to Earlswood to teach handicrafts in Bridge House and the remainder of the school classes moved to the main hospital building. Mrs. Cunningham left to become Head Teacher at

Leybourne Grange, to be replaced by Miss Smith in about 1945. However, she died two years later and Mrs. Wells returned to take over.

In 1938 there were 75 pupils in the Boys School and 23 boys and 39 girls in the mixed school, including eight of each gender in the senior class. There were 111 in the boys' continuation school. This was an intermediate stage between school and work. The intention was to prepare the youngsters for employment and so the lessons were designed to develop technical or manufacturing skills. The boys were taught to make envelopes and paper bags. Other products were woollen mats, brushes, baskets and cane-work including trays and chairs. The low-grade patients were taught bed making, brass polishing and general cleaning. On special frames they were taught how to tie and lace. All the pupils had physical drill and other physical education included punch ball, basketball, skittles, quoits and cycle riding. Musical instruments were enjoyed by all, especially the percussion band.

The school continued to supervise the correspondence of the boys and men. During 1938 there were 3487 letters, cards and papers delivered to the male patients and a complete record of the contents was kept, including postal orders, stamps etc. There were 4621 letters and cards written by and for the residents.

In 1947 the boys' continuation school was reorganised into two departments with two teachers to each. By 1950 the mixed school occupied two large rooms in the west wing of the main building. The children attended until the age of 16. They were taught by four teachers and used a technique developed by Montessori and McDouall. There were 54 pupils who were resident within Royal Earlswood and four day-pupils. The pupils studied reading, writing, arithmetic, eurhythmics, puppetry and hand bell ringing. Lessons also included lacing, buttoning, threading beads, raffia work, educational toys, jigsaws and singing games. The boys' continuation school had 65 pupils studying reading, writing and arithmetic, but also learning weaving, rug making, chair caning, envelope making, case sheet folder making and carpentry.

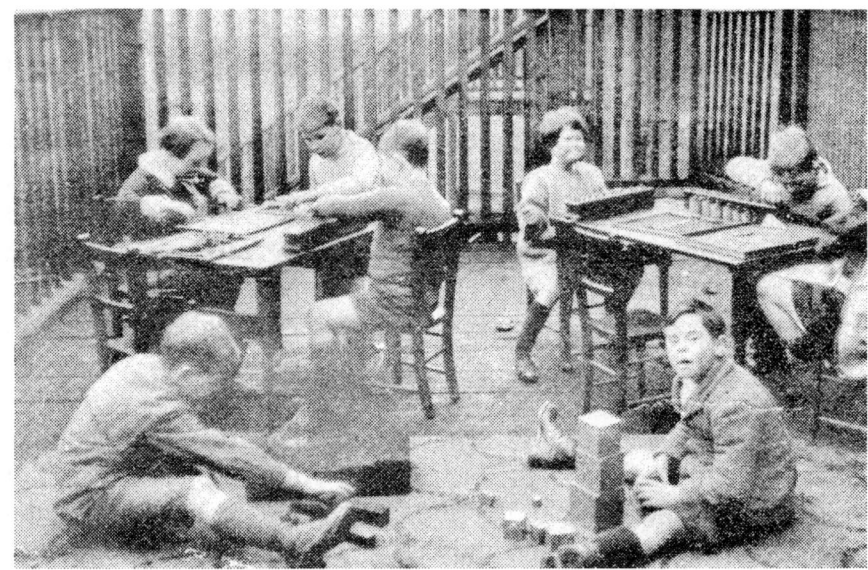

A Montessori class

In 1952 the mixed school had 55 pupils in four classes. The male continuation school had 71 pupils learning weaving, basket making, raffia weaving, stool seating and making rugs, lampshades, envelopes, case sheet folders and socks. They worked in the garden growing sufficient flowers for all the wards to have a regular supply. The boys would help on the farm lifting potatoes and during harvest time. They played cricket and football for recreation. In

Bridge House, the handicraft school provided for 54 girls over 16 years of age. They made rugs and soft toys, embroidered items, knitted jumpers, cardigans and dish clothes, operated stocking knitting machines and sewing machines. In one year they made 826 sheets, 1200 towels, 675 bath towels, 348 aprons plus 200 brush and comb bags making the Asylum self sufficient in these items and giving a surplus to sell, raising valuable revenue.

In 1957, as an experiment, the more severely learning disabled pupils were given periods of free play. These were found to be very beneficial. The nursery had a session in the morning, with older pupils between two and four o'clock in the afternoon. The children were given opportunities to play with plasticine, construction toys, musical toys etc. They each enjoyed sessions of physical training and musical activities once a week. Pupils with behaviour problems had a specially constructed playroom and had access to clay, sand and water.

In 1959 there were 62 pupils in the special school and 72 in the boys' continuation school. Occupational therapy was encouraged for the lower grade boys. Sixty-two young women attended the Bridge House Occupational Therapy Unit. About a fifth of them attended for half days and the rest were full-time students. They produced a variety of good quality handicrafts.

In 1967 work started on a new school to replace the old one, now considered to be rather inadequate and outdated. It was designed to provide education for 84 children between five and sixteen years of age. There were also teachers who worked on the wards for those children who were unable to attend. There were seven classrooms, a staff-room and offices surrounding a purpose built hall. The school was part of the new children's complex of residential accommodation at the western end of the site. An engineering plant in the school supplied the whole complex. The school was opened in 1968. It was maintained by the Hospital. However, in 1971 the responsibility for staffing the school was taken over by Surrey County Council Education Department and they rented the building from the Health Authority. Specialised modern teaching methods were introduced. Mrs. Moore was the head teacher.

The school has 70 special needs children aged from six to 19, all resident within Royal Earlswood. Additional children would attend the school for short periods whilst at Earlswood for respite care. The children suffered from a numbers of conditions including neurological problems, epilepsy, autism, sensory disability and multiple handicaps. They were divided into eight classes; seven in the school building and the eighth occupied the Andrew Reed Unit, situated in the main hospital building. This latter catered for children with hyper kinesis and psychosis. The seven classes provided a special care unit and nursery unit, together with three classes for more able children and two for older, less able children who had severe behavioural problems. The staff consisted of a head teacher and deputy, eight assistant teachers, six welfare assistants and a part-time secretary.

In some ways the pattern of education had not changed much over the intervening century. Classes included physical education and country dancing, practice with buying selling and handling money, art, cookery, swimming and the school still had a percussion band. The aims of the school were to maximise the potential of the individual child and, using realistic programs, to promote social competence, emotional development and communication.

SCHOOLMASTER'S REPORT. 1869

The number of pupils under instruction at the present time is 146.

Seventeen attend both morning and afternoon; 129 attend either morning or afternoon but not both.

During the past years 45 pupils have been received into the School. These, having a very small amount of intellectual power, have, in most cases, been placed in the lower classes. During the same period 53 pupils have left the school. Some of these have been discharged, several have died, and the remainder now devote their whole time to some useful occupation. Most of these have improved, some to a considerable extent.

The School is still divided into six classes, according to the mental attainments of the pupils. Each class receives three lessons (the morning and afternoon arrangements being nearly the same).

The subjects taught are, - Reading, Writing, Arithmetic, Shopkeeping, Drawing, telling the time by the clock, besides speaking, deaf and dumb signs, learning their own names, dressing etc. Between each of these lessons the whole of the pupils are collected in one room, and receive drilling, singing, and other collective lessons.

The mental condition of the pupils now under instruction will be shown by the following statistics:-

SPEAKING.
64 can speak fairly;
36 can speak indistinctly;
30 can make a few sounds only;
16 who do not speak at all
146

READING.
20 can read fairly;
20 can read by spelling the words;
16 know nearly all the letters;
39 know a few letters;
51 know none of the letters;
146

WRITING.
22 can write sentences in copy books;
20 can write easy words;
21 can make a few letters;
52 can make strokes and the letter O;
31 can scribble or make no attempt;
146

ARITHMETIC.
7 can do small sums by themselves:-
       1 in fractions;
       6 in the simple rules.
20 can add from blackboard, and count above a hundred;
20 can count above fifty;
18 can count above twenty-five;
53 can count a little;
28 not at all.
146

DRAWING AND IMITATION.
2 can draw on paper, with shading;
10 can draw on paper, outline only;
36 on slate, with moderate correctness;
66 can make letters with imitation frames;
32 cannot imitate.
146

SHOP LESSON.
24 know all the coins, weights, and can calculate a little;
23 know all the coins and some weights;
23 know a few coins and weights;
29 know a few coins only;
47 know none.
146

CLOCK LESSON.
8 can tell the time to the minute;
8 can tell the hours and five minutes;
12 can tell the hours;
14 can tell some of the hours;
5 know 12 o'clock;
99 not at all.
146

COLOUR LESSON.

24 know all the colours;
50 know one or two colours;
72 know none.
146

During the dark evenings, in addition to the New Year's Entertainment, several Concerts have been given, all of which have been a source of great gratification to the pupils. At these Entertainments about 60 of the officers and servants, and one or two patients take part, either vocally or instrumentally.

SCHOOLMISTRESS'S REPORT

During the past year 40 fresh cases have been admitted into the School.

Number discharged, 8 (term having expired); 2 have been removed to household work; 7 have been transferred to the Boys' School; and 7 have died.

The total number now attending school is 145, including 18 male infants.

Of this number 68 are present both morning and afternoon, and 77 in the morning only.

NEEDLEWORK
11 hem and sew well;
18 hem very fairly;
34 hem indifferently;
6 can do fancy work;
76 cannot work at all
145

MEALS
66 can use knife and fork;
24 can use a spoon and fork;
48 can use a spoon;
7 are fed
145

I am happy to state that the foregoing statistics show a decided improvement upon the last Report of 1868, thus convincing those to whose care they are entrusted that their labours are not in vain. A large proportion of those receiving instruction are very affectionate, which stimulates us to further exertion on their behalf. Generally speaking, they are well-behaved; and an approving smile from their teacher accomplishes much. The Monday evening amusements (which are eagerly anticipated throughout the week) afford extreme pleasure to one and all.

SPEAKING
48 speak fairly;
34 speak indistinctly;
28 only make sounds;
35 do not speak at all;
145

READING
16 read very fairly;
28 by spelling the words;
34 know some of the letters;
67 know none of the letters;
145

WRITING.
13 write in copy-books;
10 write copies on slates;
26 write letters on slates;
54 form strokes and O;
42 have no idea whatever;
145

ARITHMETIC.
6 work simple sums;
6 from the blackboard fairly;
15 name at sight figures up to 20;
4 count to 100 accurately;
17 to 100 by giving the tens;
29 count a little;
68 cannot count at all.
145

School reports from Annual Report 1869.

There were twelve weeks of holidays annually, but these were staggered to allow the school to remain open for 43 weeks per year, the longest break being a fortnight in August. The lessons included horse riding. There was an adventure playground and the children went camping in the grounds. Coach outings were also a regular part of the curriculum. Varied training was offered and the older children had opportunities for work experience.

The school worked closely with the Hospital. Multidisciplinary reviews were held monthly, involving the doctors, teachers, psychologists, social workers, speech therapists, physiotherapists, ward staff and parents. The school provided a training opportunity for student and pupil nurses and for student teachers. Pupils at the local comprehensive schools, who were taking their Childcare Certificate, spent time working at the school.

When the school eventually closed, the education of the learning disabled moved into the community, as for the general population. The Ellen Terry and Brooklands School, as it was then known, opened in Reigate in about 1975.

Entertainment.

The Board was determined to improve the quality of life for those given into their charge. It was not sufficient to provide board, education and occupation. They wanted to provide experiences of a more enjoyable type. Therefore, the entertainment and enlightenment of the pupils was given careful consideration. In 1865, The *'London Mirror'* reported that "The amusements of summer and winter months have been carried out with much spirit." There were monthly concerts during the winter and these were reportedly much enjoyed by the residents. "The love of music is almost universal among the inmates, and the efforts of the staff…have been amply rewarded by the delight which they have been able to inspire."

By 1869, Earlswood hosted an evening entertainment every Monday during the winter months. These included concerts, plays, minstrel shows and other popular attractions. In his report in March of that year the Medical Superintendent, George Grabham, alluded to the "brilliant display of 'Electric Fireworks' gratuitously given by Mr. Thomas Hooker." The brass band, made up of male staff from the Asylum, performed twice a week for the patients. Dr. Grabham was pleased to report the enlargement of the band and the acquisition of new instruments, procured from Paris without expense to the Institution. There was also an orchestral band, similarly composed of staff, which played regularly. In 1874 a 'drum and fife band' was reported to be doing well. On dry days during the summer months, the band would perform in

---

Schedule of Entertainment for 1866.

Annual fete
Entertainment Day (Jan)
Every Monday – one hour long entertainment
Three concerts through the year for principle inhabitants
11 Brass and string band concerts.
15 Games and band
13 Choral Union
4 Concerts
2 Punch and Judy Shows
3 Magic lantern shows
1 Bonfire with fireworks
3 Shows.

An example of the entertainment provided during one year.

the grounds on Wednesday afternoons. Some of the younger residents would take the opportunity to practice their dancing. The quadrille was apparently very popular. Tea would be taken on the lawn. Sometimes concert parties or 'strolling players' would visit the Asylum to entertain the residents. On other occasions the staff would get up a play. Even the medical staff was prepared to take a part or contribute to the concert parties.

There were processions around the ground, headed by the band. The old custom of 'beating the bounds' was practised at Earlswood. Originally a way of establishing and reinforcing ownership of an area of land the practise later took on a more symbolic role. On the 17th of July 1865 the ceremony was curtailed by the weather;

> **"Bounds were to have been beaten today but the weather being unfavourable the Committee only marched with the pupils and the brass band to the woods."**

The following year the weather did not interfere with proceedings. The band marched round the boundary of the estate with the steward, Mr. Brown, at the head. The committee and, finally, the pupils carrying flags followed them. The procession started at 12 noon and arrived back at 1.30pm.

In summer an unmanned hot air balloon was sent up once a month. There were balloon races; a report of one such event describes round balloons, together with others shaped like a fish, an ox and an elephant. Cricket matches were held regularly and these were reported in the local paper. Opponents included the Philanthropic Society.

In the winter months there were Punch and Judy shows, put on by an attendant. Magic lantern shows were also popular. They would show 'dissolving views' fifteen feet in diameter. A 'aphengerscope' was also very amusing. The board members and others gave slides. A wide variety of entertainment was available to the residents including 'glee singers', a concert party, and a dramatic company as well as the brass band and orchestra.

Guy Fawkes day was also enjoyed by the residents as everyone dressed up. There was a huge bonfire followed by a fireworks display. Mr. Halfpenny, the carpenter, constructed a wooden framework and, to this were attached, five pounds worth of Brocks fireworks – a princely sum. The following report was written by a resident at the time:

> **"First thing in the morning, November 5th, old Billy S.... got a lovely white beard he had, used to sit in the carpenter's shop. He was an expert at flying a kite. In his spare time he used to come out and sit under a tree, and he had a tremendous great kite. He used to sit under this tree and let it go up. And do you know, he used to fly this kite right over Redhill. Used to have miles and miles of cord.**
>
> **Well, in those days, they used to set off about half past nine, all dressed up, and old Billy S.... – they did look some guys too! Used to have a tremendous great guy and they would go all round, into the schools and then down Princes Road, and they would dance and sing and go all round the district."**

From 1878 onwards, evening parties were regularly held in the girls' schoolroom. These gave the young people the opportunity to experience the sorts of entertainment that would have been common in ordinary Victorian homes at the time, dancing, charades and games. There were Punch and Judy shows and games such as bagatelle.

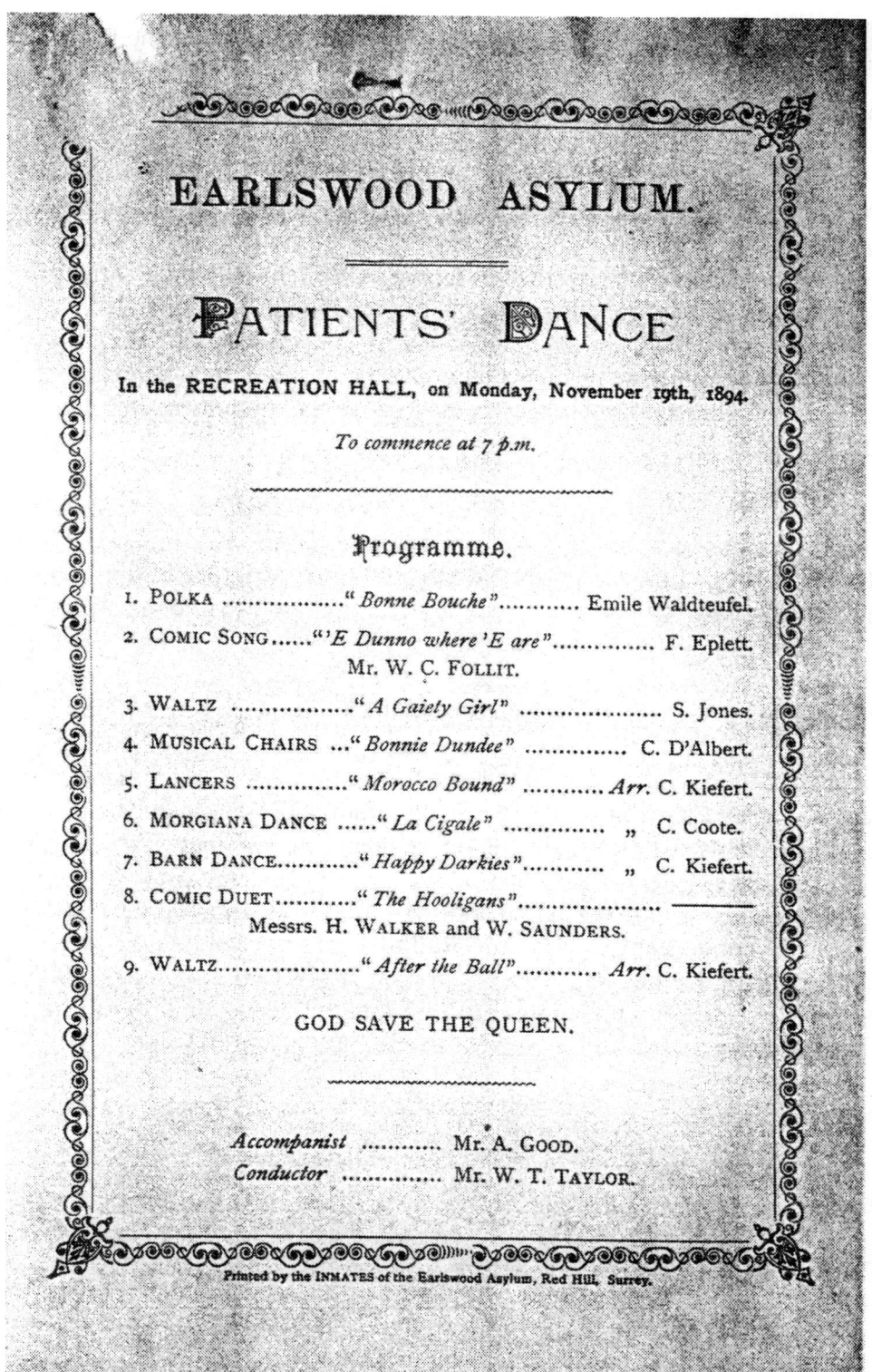

Program for a patients' dance

Entertainment was also provided for the staff. On the 15th of November 1866 Dr. Down engaged a Mr. Cockrill, for the fee of a guinea, to give a literary entertainment in the hall. Officers and attendants were invited to attend for the sum of two pence (1p) each. A pound was collected.

In 1891, The *'Earlswood Magazine'*, printed by residents themselves, gives some idea of the how the hours were spent at the Asylum. The autumn had been excessively damp, curtailing the football fixtures, but it was hoped that this would soon alter. In the meantime the indoor activities had provided diversion. A concert program had included Gilbert and Sullivan, military band music, comic songs and recitations. A harvest festival had been held on the 4th of October with decorations, texts and hymns. About one hundred and eighty people attended a dance on the 12th of October, "the children thoroughly entering into the fun of the evening." On the 19th of that month, Dr. Jones entertained all with a magic lantern tour of Belgium, Germany and Switzerland. The "most enjoyable and laughable" evening had been on the 26th of October when staff and patients joined together in a program of shadow pantomime, including "war steeds, tournaments, mephistophelian manoeuvres and the famed Blondin donkey."

In June 1906 visitors found the residents enjoying the music of the attendants' band playing in the grounds "like a garden party". They remarked on the enjoyment that was obvious in the faces of the residents, their expressions usually so vacant.

In the 1950s and 1960s a further form of entertainment was available for some of the residents of Earlswood. A pony was purchased from the International League for the Protection of Horses. Her name was Daisy and she gave rides to the children, providing a new sense of independence for those who were wheelchair bound. In 1961 Daisy was returned to the 'League' in part exchange for a chestnut gelding called Sandy. The new pony stood at fifteen and a half hands and had a flaxen mane and white socks on the hind legs. Priced at £35, Earlswood paid £12-10s (£12.50) for Sandy with the allowance given for the return of Daisy.

In 1979 Ronald Moon, charge nurse of Farm Villa, introduced a Shetland pony called Sara Jane. There was also a parrot called Pip, an aquarium and a dog named Lofty, who could be trusted to take residents out for a walk and return them safely to the ward.

Football remained a very popular game and the Earlswood team was successful. In 1957 the Hospital team became champions of the Redhill and District League Division I and was promoted to the Premier League. The evening entertainment continued until the closure of Earlswood. In 1960 the annual report records that concerts, film shows and whist drives occurred at least twice a week during the winter months.

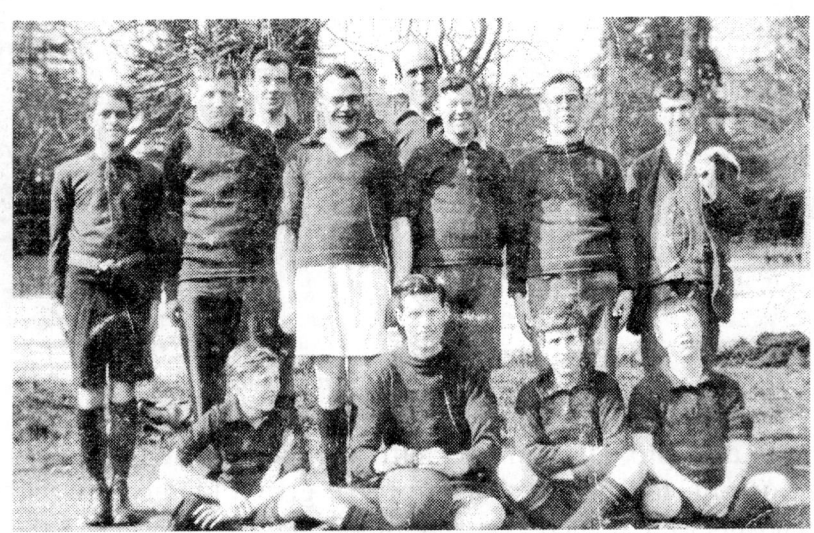

The football team

In July 1973 the Gateway Club was founded. This was initially held fortnightly in the Circle Club building within the Hospital grounds. In February 1974 the club was affiliated to the

National Federation of Gateway Clubs. The aim of the club was to integrate the children resident within the Hospital with those in the community at large. Initially 25 children attended it from Earlswood and five from outside. Ten children from Brooklands School soon joined them.

Training

An early report from the inspectors criticised the absence of useful employment, especially for the boys at Earlswood. Funding was needed for the purchase of gardening implements, materials for making straw hats, bonnets and mats and the provision of small animals for the study of animal husbandry. However, these omissions were soon rectified and by 1862 the Commissioners in Lunacy reported that 95% of the residents were benefiting from useful occupation.

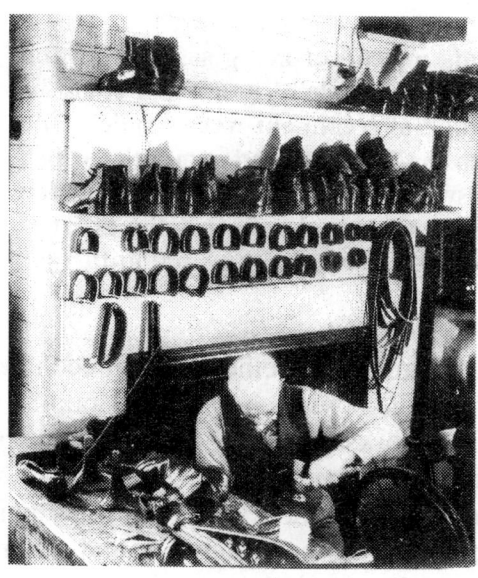

Boot and shoe shop

Training was a major element of the treatment offered at Earlswood; the first institution in Britain so organised. Only those who were felt to be capable of benefiting from training were to be admitted. However, in an effort to avoid excluding a person inappropriately the aim from the earliest days was a balance composed of 25% of residents who were very able, 50% fairly able and 25% who may be capable of only slight improvement. If any proved incapable of improvement they would be ineligible for re-election at the end of their initial period at the Asylum.

Annual reports contained illustrations of what could be achieved.

> **"E.B., a girl, aged twenty years. Admitted, *October*, 1849. A few months since she commenced assisting one of the nurses, but proved at first rather a hindrance; she could not be left alone for a moment, could not sweep, dust or scrub. *April* 1853. The nurse now states that she is a great help; everything is now properly arranged; she can sweep, dust and scrub nicely. Her countenance is more cheerful and intelligent, and the silliness of manner she had for a long time after her admission is passing away."**

> **"S.P., a girl, aged thirteen years. Admitted, *May*, 1850. A congenital Idiot; had a peculiar drawl in her speech, which was almost inarticulate; had a vacant look and an awkward gait; was very feeble and could not write. *April*, 1853. Her**

81

speech is greatly improved, so that she can be distinctly understood; she is stronger in mind and body, reads and writes well, is very useful with her needle, and has the charge of one of the bed-rooms."

The staffing levels at the Asylum were very low and the view was taken that the residents should be encouraged, as far as possible, to care for themselves and those less able. In the early days many were discharged so improved that they were able to find employment. Ten percent became self-supporting whilst 40% gained useful employment and, if not totally independent, they were at least able to contribute to the family income. Forty-four percent were significantly improved and only six percent were not improved. In 1865 one shoemaker reputedly left Earlswood as a journeyman, able to make six pairs of boots a week.

In February 1866 a Northern Asylum was planned to run on the same lines as Earlswood. *'The Sheffield Independent'* reported:

> **"At Earlswood it had been shown that idiots instead of being so helpless and hopeless as to be incapable of being elevated in the scale of humanity, could be dealt with very successfully if a proper method of treatment were applied, and that their improvement was in proportion to the kindness and sympathy which was brought to bear upon them... The Earlswood Asylum would be the model; and that institution was one of the finest ornaments and reflected the greatest amount of credit upon the benevolence of the country of any philanthropic establishment."**

In 1880 it was reported that the workshops provided training, together with an economic way to make and repair articles required by the Institution. The boys' school had 91 pupils, 64 on a part-time basis. The remaining time was spent in the workshops. Boys would move between the different units until a type of work was found that was compatible with their abilities. A pupil made brushes with the help of one 'younger inmate' without supervision by paid staff. Seventeen boys were in the tailoring workshop, four each in the woodwork and shoemaker's shops, five made baskets, two were trainee printers and the remainder were in the industrial

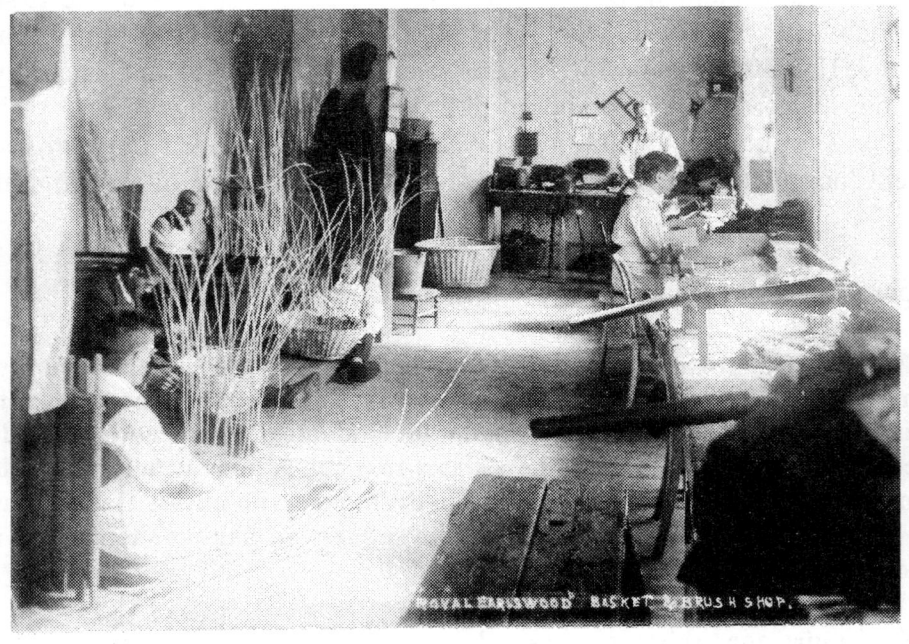

Basket and brush making shop

training unit. The training appears to have been very effective. In 1897, specimens of the girls' needlework were sold at an Arts and Crafts Exhibition in Lancaster. In a section especially for the inmates of Asylums, 17 prizes were awarded to Earlswood.

The master carpenter lamented the discharge of a former pupil who had been worth a pound a week to the Institution and demonstrated with pride the panels and doors of another who would, he said, be able to earn his living anywhere after his three years at Earlswood. Similar degrees of expertise were evident in the tailoring and shoemakers' workshops. The greatest expertise was in the Print workshop, the only one to take outside work. In addition to tasks for the Asylum and the London office over 230 orders were taken in 1898 making a profit of £150. Another discharged resident earned ten shillings (50p) a week in a grocer's shop. He belonged to a Bible class and paid into an insurance club that would guarantee his mother ten shillings and sixpence (52.5p) a week, and pay all doctors bills, in the event that he was ill. His relatives admitted that, without training, he would have been a burden to his family for his whole life.

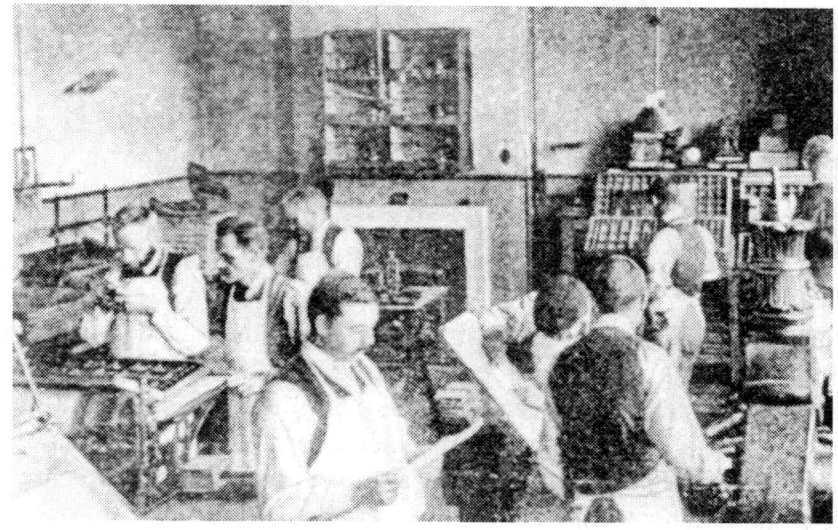

Print office

In 1906 an article in *'The Globe'* recorded that 30% of the patients in Earlswood could be taught a trade, although some supervision or control was always necessary. However, as with all young people not all pupils wanted to learn. In 1899 *'The Quiver'* reported on those who were less than willing:

> **"You can't make me work, you know, doctor,' one patient maintained, 'for I am only an imbecile."**

In 1910 at the Festival Dinner it was reported that Earlswood trained inmates to the following trades:

> **"baker, carpenter, wood-carver, fretworker, printer, compositor, shoemaker, tailor, basket, brush and mat maker, bookbinder, upholsterer, plumber, painter, farmhand, gardener, house maid, laundry maid and kitchen helper."**

In 1912 the name of the Institution was changed as the terms idiot and imbecile became less acceptable. The 'National Training Home for the Feeble-Minded' was chosen to reflect the emphasis placed on that element of care.

The same year *'The Daily Telegraph'* carried a report of the Festival Dinner in which it praised the work of the Asylum. Five thousand people had received training by this time, 500 were currently benefiting. One man had left Earlswood after 18 years and was sufficiently improved that he was able to earn his living in Johannesburg, possibly his family home as many residents were accepted from abroad. Another, after 10 years, had been accepted into a British regiment and had fought in the Boer War.

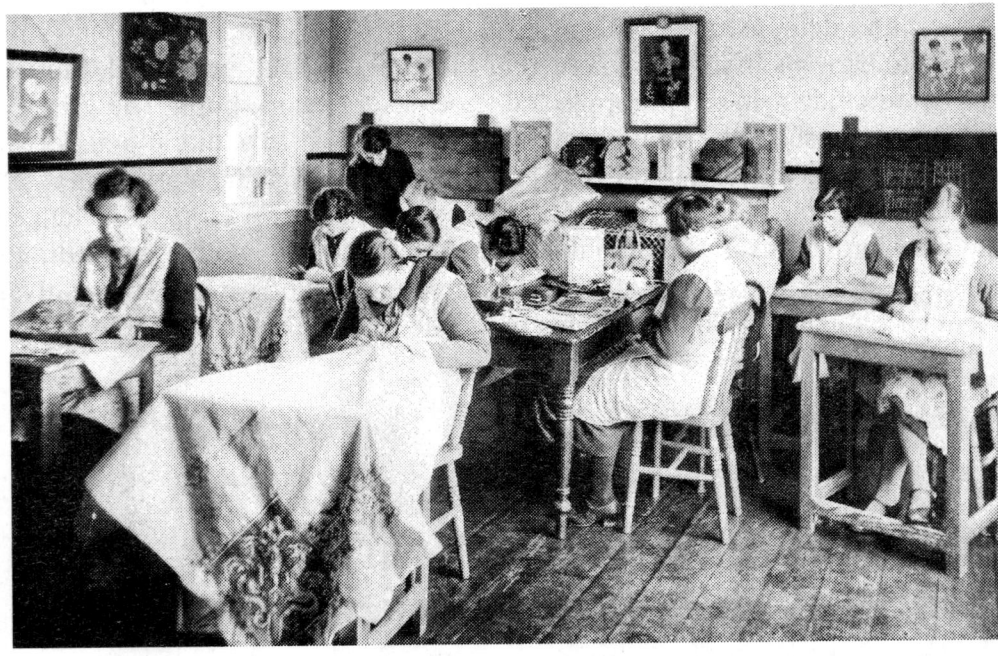

Needlework shop

In 1952 the annual report recorded that there were 54 girls over the age of 16 years being trained in a variety of skills, rug making, embroidery, knitting, soft toy making and the use of sewing or stocking making machines. The older boys attended the male continuation school where they produced baskets, raffia work, woven items, socks, stool seating, rugs, lampshades, envelopes, cases and sheet folders. They grew sufficient flowers for all the wards and helped on the farm during harvest and potato lifting. They played cricket and football for exercise and to develop team spirit.

In 1965 a new supervisor took over the Occupational Therapy department. It was accommodated at the time in the dilapidated Bridge House, with coal fires, bare floors and depressing décor. Forty-five female patients worked there with three instructors, making rugs and other handicraft items. The building had been condemned and a new one was planned.

A programme of industrial work was introduced in the morning, with handicrafts and cookery sessions in the afternoon. The success of the programme was such that it quickly became clear that the planned new building would be inadequate. Bridge House was modernised and used for social training whilst the new unit, named the Anderson Centre after a previous medical superintendent, was finished two years later and formed the industrial therapy unit.

The male Occupation Therapy department was housed in a block above the laundry. The roof leaked and it was impossible to keep the place clean and warm. In June 1969 the male and female departments were merged in the new building. Eventually the old garage and barn next to Bridge House were converted into studios to accommodate Art and Music Therapy. In October 1972 a purpose built industrial and occupational training unit, large enough to house both male and female clients, was opened by Sir Desmond Bonham-Carter, the Chairman of the South West Metropolitan Regional Hospital Board. Called the Thomas Parker Centre and accommodating 150 people, it liberated the smaller Anderson Centre to be converted into an

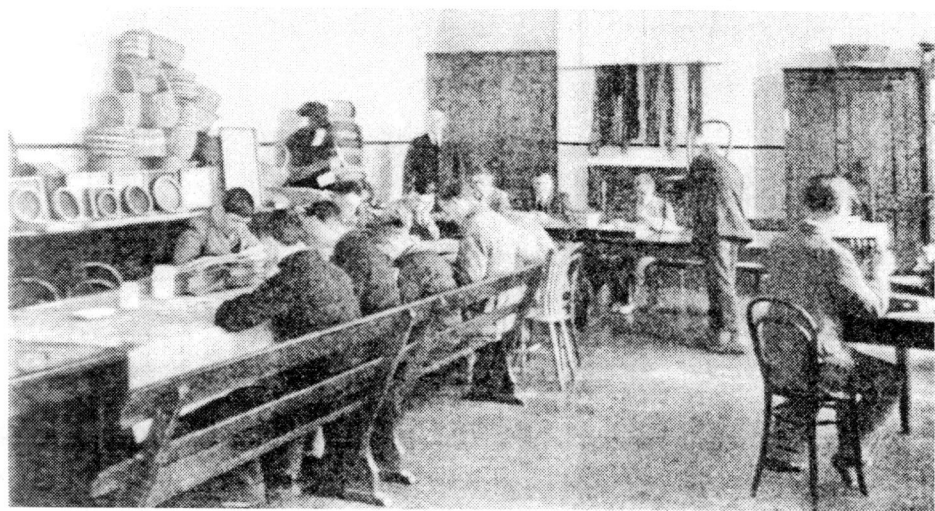

Making paper bags

Assessment and Special Care Unit. This completed the 'Department of Technical and Social Training' complex in the north west corner of the Earlswood site.

In 1973 280 people attended the new 'Technical and Social Training Department', mostly on a full-time basis. By 1977 this had risen to 300 trainees, housed in the three buildings. They were divided into 13 groups with 29 training staff, and following a varied programme over a six-week cycle. The training was designed to give every individual a balanced programme that would develop them to their maximum potential and help them to integrate into society and the workplace. The multi-disciplinary team would assess their progress regularly. The trainees received wages that they were free to spend as they wished. Those who were not capable of looking after themselves were taken on shopping expeditions or to places of entertainment. The more able were permitted to leave the Hospital alone.

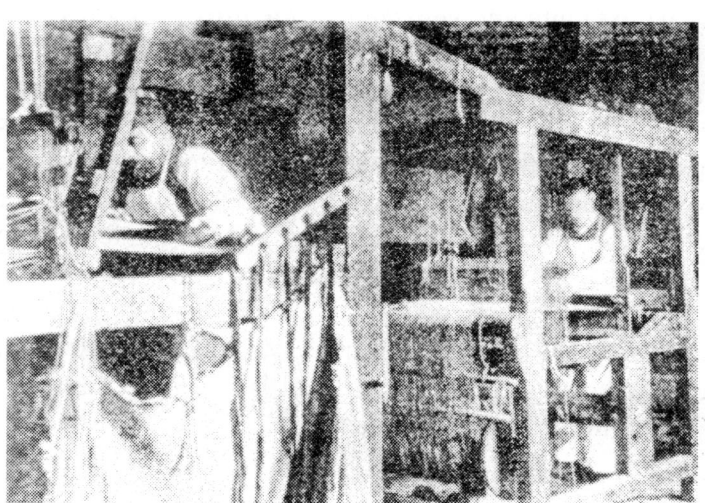

Mat making workshop

The Anderson Centre catered for those with multiple disabilities and the training concentrated on basic life skills with sweets as the reward for effort. If sufficient progress was made the trainees would transfer to the Transitional Group housed in the Parker Centre before moving finally into the formal industrial unit in that building. Designed to accommodate 150 people, this unit could accept various tasks required by outside industry, from plastic trimming and woodworking to simple and complex packaging, assembly and mailing. The trainees gained skill, and experience of the work environment, within 'safe' surroundings. There was an expectation that they would take responsibility for their work, their time keeping and their behaviour towards fellow workers.

The following subjects were provided within the training units and some sessions were also provided on the wards for those unable to attend the units:

Handicrafts – rug making, needlework, knitting and simple sewing.
Arts and crafts – group activities including collages, cane work and stool seating.
Further education – extra tuition in reading, writing and arithmetic.
Cookery and house crafts – clothes care, washing and ironing, use of household equipment, shopping.
Social training – designed to enable the adult to survive in the ordinary world the topics included assertiveness training, time, use of public transport, personal hygiene, use of the telephone, letter writing etc.
Art Therapy was available for those who would benefit from this mode of expression.
Music Therapy provided a means of communication for those often unable to express themselves well in words.
Sensory and perception, fine and gross motor skills, relaxation
Computer aided teaching.
Visiting the doctor or dentist.
Physical training included simple exercises, swimming, football, cricket and other team games.
Exercises in water were particularly pleasant for those normally confined to wheelchairs.
Medau – there was a weekly session of this specialised form of movement to music.
Drama – twice-weekly sessions led to occasional productions, but in addition, contributed much as a form of speech therapy.
Horseriding – students who attended this at a local riding school also learned about the care of the horses they rode.
Horticulture – skills were taught and vegetables were grown for the cookery sessions.

In October 1972, as a further form of training, a 'token' economy was introduced on Albert Home, one of the male wards, with residents earning tokens for shaving and bed making. These could then exchange in the Hospital shops, used to pay for attendance at a disc jockey session on Saturday afternoons or exchanged for spending money for use on holiday. The scheme worked well and was extended in February 1973 to the female hostel.

Training was not merely a formalised process. In 1967 Diana Cortazzi, the senior psychologist, started the Royal Earlswood Women's Institute. By 1969 it had 20 members. At each meeting the hymn 'Jerusalem' was sung. Members of local W.I. groups came to help the residents. All were involved in making the Institution banner.

Medical staff

When the Society was first founded one member of the Board was the already distinguished Dr. W J Little (1810-94). He had joined the staff of the London Hospital in 1839 and had published a description of spastic diplegia, later known as Little's disease, before becoming involved with the Charity. He continued to work as one of the honorary medical officers for Earlswood until 1889 and, in addition, founded the Orthopaedic Infirmary, now the Royal National Orthopaedic Hospital.

A second member of the Board, and honorary medical officer, from the beginning was Dr. John Conolly (1794-1866). Born in Market Rasen, Lincolnshire, he was the orphaned son of an Irishman. He attended grammar school in Hedon until he was nine years old. In 1803 his mother married a Frenchman who taught him his native tongue. At 18 he joined the militia, he later married and moved to France. Returning to Britain around 1817 or 1818 he entered medical school at the University of Edinburgh, completing his degree in 1821. He set up in practice in Chichester but due to the low income he decided to apply for the post of Medical Superintendent at Hanwell Lunatic Asylum, county asylum for Middlesex. Rejected at his first attempt in 1838, he was finally appointed in 1839. This gave him an entrée into London society. He used his new influence to speak out against the use of restraint in treatment.

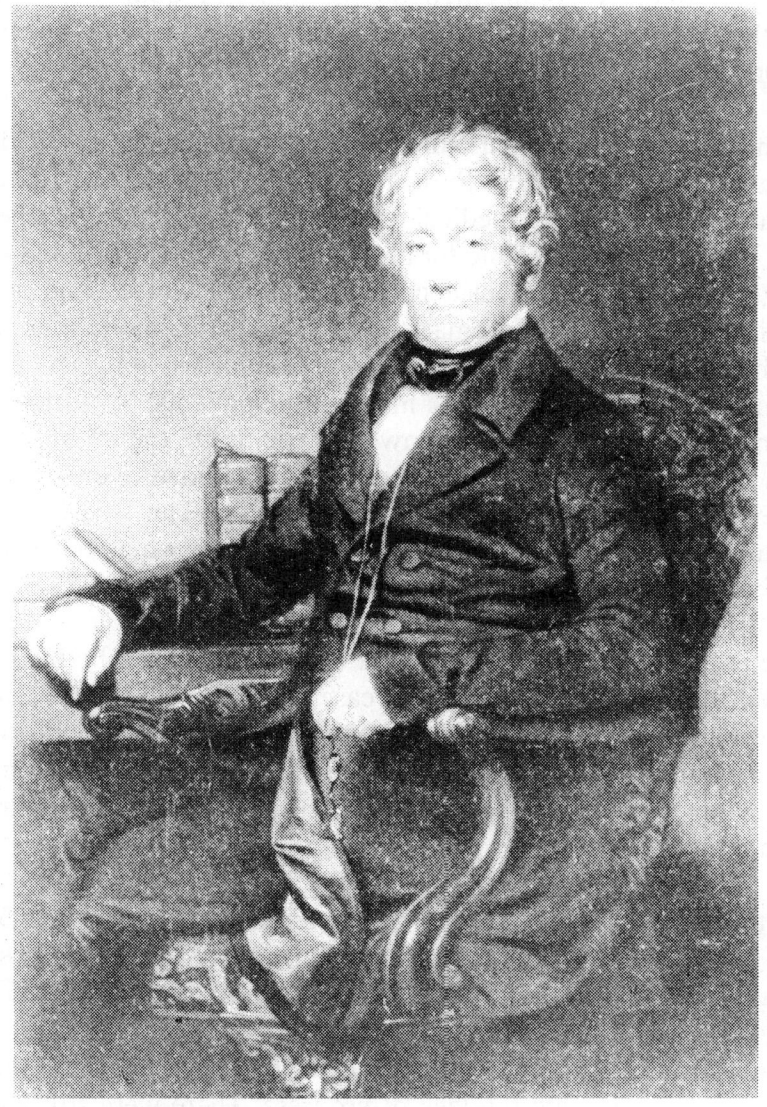

Dr. John Conolly

(Reprinted with the permission of the Royal College of Physicians)

As honorary physician to the Charity he was influential in determining the conditions at the Asylum and the methods of treatment used. Having discontinued the use of constraint within Hanwell Lunatic Asylum, he was keen to repeat the experiment. In the first ten years there were only a handful of cases when restraint was used. Restraint was only considered necessary when an inmate's behaviour represented a risk to themselves or others. One recorded case was to prevent the "swallowing of stones and filth" and another to stop a resident from "producing sickness" by constantly putting her hands down her throat.

By 1874 the use of mechanical restraint was limited to the wearing of leather or woollen gloves to prevent children from picking or injuring their hands. Leather gloves were fitted around the wrists and were worn at night for surgical reasons or by patients who had "mischievous or destructive propensities". Records show that leather gloves were employed for periods from two to seven weeks but in twenty months this form of restraint was used only five times and by 1881 was employed only for surgical reasons. Restraint had been completely abolished by 1896.

Dr. Conolly also believed that nursing required personal and intellectual skills rather than brute force and a strong nerve. Attendants were not allowed to use physical violence and the Commissioners in Lunacy frequently commented on the superior quality of the staff at Earlswood. In May 1877 they reported that the nurses and attendants were intelligent and took a great interest in their work.

For most of Earlswood's history the medical superintendent was responsible for the day-to-day operation of the Asylum. However, when Park House was first opened the role of superintendent was separate from that of the medical officer. The former post was held be Mr. Millard whilst Dr. R.C. Foreman was responsible for all medical matters. Appointed in October 1848, at a salary of 200 guineas per annum plus accommodation for himself and one servant, the latter proved less than satisfactory. Dr. Foreman failed to adopt the modern approach and continued to employ mechanical restraints. In late 1849 he introduced a "powerful electrifying machine" that he felt would be beneficial in treating many of the patients. No further reference is made to this and it seems unlikely that he was allowed to use it. On the 8th of April 1850 a special meeting was held to look into his conduct. He was reprimanded over several matters and resigned later that month after less than two years of office. The Board accepted his resignation whilst recording their appreciation of the enthusiasm with which he "had attended to the interests of the Institution and to the welfare of the patients therein".

The medical officers were required to adhere to a number of rules laid down by the Board. The medical superintendent had immediate authority in the case of emergencies. However, he had to answer for his actions to the House Committee. Amongst his other responsibilities he was required to gather evidence of the benefits derived by the residents from the benevolent treatment offered at the Asylum. He was also to ensure that the children were never at any time left in want of supervision.

Dr. Maxwell was the next medical superintendent to be appointed but initially the Board only granted him a temporary position at four guineas per week in order to assess his suitability. After one month he was given a contract for a year. He stayed until September 1858, moving with the patients to Earlswood in 1855. During Dr. Maxwell's eight-year term of office the number of residents increased from 70 to 205. A deficiency of funds led the Commissioners of Lunacy to express their dissatisfaction with the lack of progress. There were still a number of problems with the building such as the lack of night staff and the condition of the drinking water as detailed previously. Furthermore the Commissioners of Lunacy complained that statutory records were entirely neglected and urged the medical superintendent to adhere to the *"Act for the Regulation for the Care and Treatment of Lunatics, 1845"*, relating to the keeping of records. Every incorrect item or omission rendered the medical superintendent liable to a fine of £20. In 1858 Dr. Maxwell resigned and the Commissioners recommended that an additional sum be identified to increase the medical superintendent's salary from the inadequate level of 250 guineas per annum.

Dr. J. Langdon-Down (1828-96) replaced Dr. Maxwell and received the much-improved sum of £400 per annum, together with furnished accommodation, coal and gas. This was increased to £600 in 1864 and then by £50 in each of the next two years.

Dr. Down was born in Torpoint, Cornwall in 1828, the youngest of six children, and left school at thirteen to work with his father who was an apothecary. He moved to London in 1846 and he was apprenticed to an apothecary, Matthew Coleman, at 265 Whitechapel Road. He enrolled as a student at the Pharmaceutical Society in Bloomsbury Square. The skills he gained would have equipped him to develop medicines that his father could sell. There he assisted Faraday in some of his experiments on gases. Unfortunately, he became ill and had to spend three years in Devon recuperating. He resumed his scientific career in London teaching chemistry but was recalled to Devon by his father's illness and death in 1853. A long-term drink problem may have contributed to his father's death, explaining Down's subsequent belief in the dangers of alcohol.

Financially supported by his sister's husband, he then enrolled at the London Hospital Medical School. There he was to work with Dr. William Little who was an advisor at Earlswood. Down graduated second in his class, receiving the gold medal for physiology. Intelligent and hard working, Down 'accumulated' qualifications. These included an initial degree and MB degree from the University of London; he was a Licentiate of Worshipful Society of Apothecaries, Member of the Royal College of Surgeons and Resident in Obstetrics. There followed an MD from the University of London and Membership of the Royal College of Physicians in the year after he took up the post at Earlswood.

He was appointed to the post of Medical Superintendent in 1859. He was also elected assistant physician at the London Hospital and ultimately rose to the post of lecturer in the Principles and Practices of Medicine. Down's sister and brother-in-law agreed to move to Earlswood with him to run his household. They paid for their own accommodation and furnished it themselves. They even subsidised a stall at the annual fund-raising bazaar.

In October 1860 Down married Mary Crellin, sister to his brother-in-law. They had two children during their time at Earlswood, Everleigh in 1862 and Lilian in 1863. Tragically Lilian died following a seizure in 1865 and Everleigh died following a tragic accident in 1883 in which his brother Reginald, born in 1866, was implicated.

Down was a strict disciplinarian and staff members were dismissed for no worse crime than being out late. In particular, he would tolerate no ill treatment of the residents and several of the nursing staff were dismissed for roughness. In April 1859 he reduced staff numbers but improved the quality of staff appointed by increasing the wages. He abolished staggered lunches. The residents all ate at 12.30pm and the staff at 1.15pm. Staff started work earlier. They were no longer issued with rations to be eaten anywhere but were to take their meals in the dining hall. The attendants' beer ration was reduced to one pint per day and it was available to residents only when authorised by the Medical Superintendent. However, he provided unlimited port for the Board members!!

Down was granted permission to carry out post mortem examinations following all deaths, where possible, and by 1861 had completed 100 in total. Great progress was made at the Institution during his time as medical superintendent and staff turnover decreased. Within three months of his appointment the Commissioners commented with pleasure on the improvements that had been achieved. Down had responsibility for the running of the entire establishment and he was required to publish a report annually on the progress of the Asylum. The Institution was growing steadily, and so was the workload for the medical superintendent. In 1865 the first assistant medical officer was appointed with a salary of £100 per annum.

George Shuttleworth was a useful addition. In 1867 he assisted Down when, together with Fletcher Beach and William Ireland, two doctors dedicated to the study of Learning Disability, he co-organised the first conference on Idiocy held in Belfast. Ultimately Shuttleworth left Earlswood to become Medical Superintendent of the Northern Counties (Royal Albert) Asylum near Lancaster.

During his time at Earlswood Dr. Down began to investigate a theory that he had formulated regarding the connection between physical characteristics and types of mental disorder. He instituted the policy of taking photographs of all residents. These theories were first mentioned in 1866 in a paper *'Observations on an Ethnic Classification of Idiots'*. Initially he divided all clients into four types that he defined by racial features – Mongolian, Ethiopian, Caucasian, and American Indian. Only one of these groups ultimately proved of lasting interest, that exhibiting the 'Mongolian' features. Once identified with the term mongolism, the genetic disorder became generally known as Downs Syndrome in 1961. Down finally published a definitive description in 1887 in a monograph, *'Mental Afflictions of Childhood and Youth'*. Down may also have been the first to describe Prader Willi Syndrome.

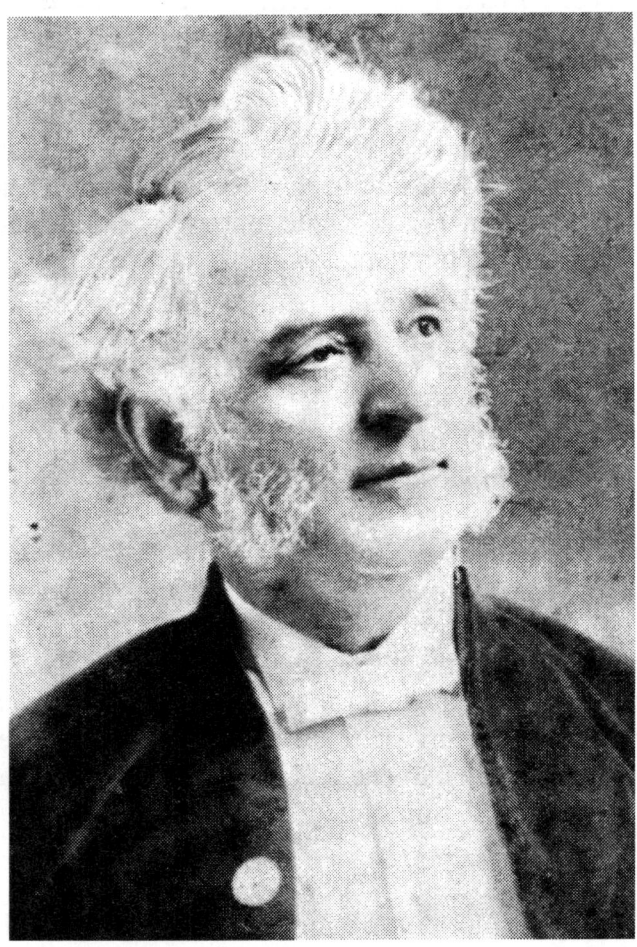

(Reprinted with the permission of the Royal College of Physicians)

Dr. John Haydon Langdon Down

Dr. Down believed in training for the learning disabled and implemented this policy at Earlswood. Two-thirds of the children were taught in the school for at least ten hours per week.

There was one care worker for every three residents. He encouraged self-sufficiency on the estate; even the sewage was used on the farm. He was safety conscious; a safety key was used to control all hot water taps. There were weekly concerts, an orchestra and band were established and an organ appeal launched. The residents sang grace before and after every meal. Cricket was played every Wednesday and Saturday, a mile of walks was developed within the grounds and 6000 trees were planted. He was very well respected and was awarded a Fellowship of the Royal College of Physicians in 1868.

Down left Earlswood in 1868 but the manner of his leaving was somewhat unusual. In January 1868 a Special Sub-Committee of the House Committee of Earlswood had cause to question the remuneration of two attendants as it exceeded that normally paid. Dr. Down was called upon to explain the additional sum being received by the two men. It transpired that the wives of the two attendants had charge of a number of patients at the suggestion of Dr. Down himself. The women were themselves under the care and supervision of Mrs. Down. Dr. Down also reported that there were a number of other persons lodged in houses unconnected with the Asylum, also under the management of Mrs. Down. Dr. Down explained that he felt the arrangement to be beneficial as it "conserved the interests of the Institution by preserving desirable patients for forthcoming vacancies"'. He also felt it to be reasonable that the women be allowed, in this way, to supplement their husband's income.

The Sub-Committee wrote to request further information from Dr. Down on the matter. This included the number and names of the patients, with whom they had been placed, the sum being paid for their care and to whom, what records were being kept, whether any of the cases had been turned down by Earlswood and whether Dr. Down, himself, provided any medical care. Two days later Dr. Down responded with the following words.

> **"in my ...letter to the Board, I stated with all frankness Mrs. Down's relation to the cases under her care, and was content to place the question as one of principle for the Board of Management to determine on.**
>
> **You appear, however, by the character of some of the questions to which you request replies, to desire to enter into matters of detail of a purely private nature rather than confer with me on the principle involved.**
>
> **This mode of treating the subject appears to me so indicative of your having arrived at a foregone conclusion in the matter that I must respectfully decline replying to your enquiries, and as there have been other circumstances which have led me to contemplate leaving, I have taken this opportunity of forwarding to the Board my resignation...."**

Dr. Down's resignation was not to be his last business with Earlswood, however. In June 1868 Down and two men toured the Asylum unaccompanied. Angered, the Board banned him from the premises unless permission for a visit was granted. In October 1868 the new medical superintendent, Dr. Grabham, seeking information from the records of two patients, found their entries to be missing from the general register. On further investigation it was found that 159 pages, representing the entries for 159 residents, had been cut from the register books. A letter was sent to Dr. Down asking whether he could throw any light on the matter. He replied that the Assistant Medical Officer had kept the records and that he had never removed or sanctioned the removal of any pages from the register.

The matter was considered by the Commissioners of Lunacy to be very serious. The Committee applied both to the assistant medical officer for information and the schoolmaster's son, Mr. Wood, was contacted as he had been employed by Dr. Down to transcribe some of the documents.

RULES

FOR

MEDICAL SUPERINTENDENT.

That he be resident in the Asylum.

That he be a duly registered medical practitioner, and that he have the entire supervision of the Establishment, and be responsible to the Board for its good management, economy, order, and efficiency in every department.

That he be responsible for the condition of the Asylum, and superintend the medical and moral treatment of the Inmates, subject to the rules of the Asylum and the orders of the Board of Management.

That he have full power to engage upon trial all Attendants and Servants, duly reporting such engagement to the next House Committee, who shall thereupon report the same to the next meeting of the Board of Management for confirmation and appointment ; and that he have power to suspend for misconduct all Attendants and Servants, duly reporting the circumstances of each such suspension to the House Committee at their next Meeting, who shall thereupon report the same to the next Meeting of the Board of Management for their final decision ; or, in the event of any emergency, to the Board direct.

That he see all the Inmates once in each day, and that he make a daily visit to every part of the House, and an occasional visit, early and late, to the dormitories, whilst the Inmates shall be in bed.

That he regulate the diet, clothing, exercise, occupation, and amusements of the Inmates, and encourage them to take exercise.

That he order and enforce all such means as he shall consider necessary or desirable for promoting and preserving the general health of the Inmates, and that he devise and carry out all such special measures as he may think expedient for invigorating and improving the bodily condition of the Inmates generally, and for encouraging the development of their mental powers.

That he keep the Medical Visitation Book as prescribed by Act of Parliament, and also a Case Book, in such manner as is prescribed by Act 8 and 9 Vict., c. 100, and in such form as the Commissioners in Lunacy have ordered, or as they may from time to time direct.

That he determine the general proceedings of the House, the hour of rising, the length of time to be spent in training, and the mode of training the physical and mental powers of the Inmates in exercise, occupation, amusement, and in the schoolrooms respectively.

That he keep a " Journal of Occurrences," and an account of all medicines, wines, and spirits dispensed to the Inmates.

That he report to the House Committee all cases which may be so far improved as to be fit for discharge.

That he make a General Report once a year to the Board of Management of the result of the various measures ordered or carried into effect by him, or under his orders, in reference to the Inmates or otherwise, and also of the progress and general condition of the whole establishment.

That he draw up a list of the duties of all Attendants and Servants of the Institution, and place a copy thereof in the hands of each, at the time of his or her appointment.

That he have power to call in any physician, surgeon, or any other medical practitioner, when necessary, in consultation, at the expense of the Institution.

Dr. White reported that he had noted the casebooks to be in an imperfect state when they were given into his charge when Dr. Down resigned. Mr. Wood could add nothing except the names of two other men, Barnard and Arnold who had also been employed to copy records. Mr. Barnard replied to the Committee's letter that he believed that the casebooks had been disordered at the time he was asked to copy them and that they had been incomplete for a number of years. The pages that were missing included patients who had died or been discharged between 1855 and 1864. Despite an investigation lasting four months the matter was never brought to a satisfactory conclusion.

BYE LAWS.

That in all cases of death, serious illness, or any emergency, he shall immediately communicate with the Secretary at the Office, and with the friends of the Inmate.

That he shall not absent himself without the consent of the Board or House Committee, except in cases of emergency, to be reported immediately to the Office.

That his whole time and services be at the disposal of the Board; that he be engaged at a yearly salary, to be regulated by the Board (the engagement to be subject to three months' notice on either side); and that he do not practise on his own account, or receive private pupils.

That he visit the Inmates at their daily meals.

That he have charge of such correspondence as may be required to be carried on at the Asylum, and preserve a copy of all letters written by him, on the business of the Institution, in a letter-book provided for that purpose, to be produced to the House Committee.

That all casts, photographs, official registers or journals, relative to the Inmates, or to the business or affairs of the Asylum, be provided at the expense of the Board, and remain their property.

That the names of all the persons present at the death of an Inmate be recorded, and reported by him to the House Committee.

That he present a written Report to each House Committee, and be in attendance to give any explanation that may be required, (whether at the House Committee or at the Board Meetings in Town).

That all Books and Journals kept by the Medical Superintendent be laid on the table at each House Committee meeting.

That the Book provided for recording the times of leaving and returning to the Asylum, of the Superintendent and every Officer of the Institution be regularly kept.

That the Medical Superintendent be permitted to record his absence in a separate book to be kept by himself, and to be presented by him to the Gentlemen representing the House Committee at each meeting.

That under no circumstances shall the Resident Superintendent and the Assistant Medical Officer be absent from the Asylum at the same time.

That a book be kept containing a Register of every Case admitted into the Asylum stating fully the condition of the Case on admission; and that this book be posted up weekly, stating the progress, if any, since admission, with other necessary remarks. That this book be kept in the Board-room, and the Superintendent only be allowed to take extracts from, or copies of it, without the consent of the Committee. That a similar Book or Register be kept for all patients admitted into the Hospital, to be posted up daily by the Assistant Medical Officer; and that a card be placed at the head of each Patient's bed, with the name and age of the Patient, the name of the disease, and the dietary legibly written thereon. The Books to be so kept as to furnish a complete record of all Cases in the Asylum, whereby the history, progress and present state of any Case may be ascertained at short notice.

That in every case of death occurring in the Establishment, the Superintendent be empowered to make an examination of the body, unless any objection to such a course has been previously made by the friends of the Patient.

That the Correspondence of Medical Referees be attached to the papers of the Cases to which they relate.

PRINTED BY THE INMATES OF THE EARLSWOOD ASYLUM.

After leaving Earlswood Dr. Langdon Down extended his Harley Street practice and took a large house near Kingston, set in four acres of ground. He opened a home for learning disabled children from well to do families. Normansfield, as it was called, expanded over the following years. By the late 1870's, set in forty acres of landscaped grounds with four villas and a sanatorium, the hospital accommodated 125 children and young people and 100 staff. Dr. Down suffered from severe influenza in 1890 and never fully recovered. He collapsed and died in 1896, aged 68. The hospital was managed by three generations of the Down family before being absorbed into the N.H.S. in 1952.

Dr. Grabham replaced Dr. Langdon Down in 1868. His starting salary was £500 per annum with unfurnished apartments in the Asylum. In 1870 the salary was increased to £600. Dr. Grabham held the position of medical superintendent for 14 years and further improved standards within the Institution. It proved very difficult to obtain sufficient attendants and nurses, not least because of the strict rules of employment, the lack of leisure, the poor pay and the rigors of the work that demanded great patience and kindness. Dr. Grabham recommended the appointment of married attendants and this proved a great advance. Another innovation introduced by Dr. Grabham was an industrial training school for girls. Here they were taught cooking and a range of other domestic skills.

In 1902 Dr. Caldecott, the Medical Superintendent of the time, was asked by the Board to look into a number of concerns regarding the running of the Institution, especially the financial position at the time. The Board accepted his recommendations that the Medical Superintendent should have more control of the day-to-day running of the Institution. He should have the power to hire and dismiss staff, and to discipline unsatisfactory behaviour or performance. Dr. Caldecott felt that the superintendent should have overall management of the farm and kitchen garden. He even took responsibility for ordering the meat within the Asylum, with a resulting saving of £1000 per annum. One of the recommendations that he made was that the Medical Superintendent should have two Assistant Medical Officers to allow him adequate time for other affairs within the Asylum. However, he advised that these should each be appointed for a maximum term of three years. On the other hand Dr. Caldecott expressed concern that there had been five different Medical Superintendents in the past twenty years and he wanted to improve the post in order to achieve longer tenure.

1848-1850	R C Foreman MD
1850-1858	J Maxwell LRCS
1859-1868	J Langdon Haydon Down MD
Jun 21st 1868 - Sept 4th 1882	George Wallington Grabham M.D. Lond.
Sept 20th 1882 - Apr 18th 1888	C W Cobbold MD
Apr 18th 1888 - Mar 27th 1893	R Armstrong Jones MD
Mar 27th 1893 - Jul 17th 1894	Lloyd Francis MD
Jul 18th 1894 - Sept 26th 1896	H. Corner MD
Oct 5th 1896 - Oct 14th 1923(Died)	Charles Caldecott MB, BS
Sept 15th 1923 - 1938	P S B Langton MB, BS
Apr 13th 1938 - Jul 10th 1964	H R Ferguson MB, ChB, DPM
Sept 25th 1964 - 1972	D E W Anderson MRCS, DPM. MRC Psych.
LRCP.	

List of Resident Physician, Medical Superintendents.

In 1909 the University of London recognised the hospital as suitable for training doctors prior to their Mental Diseases examinations. In July 1910 Dr. Pearce, the senior Assistant Medical Officer left the Asylum. A presentation was made. In January 1911 the Assistant Medical Superintendent was Dr. Nelson. In July that year Dr. Caldecott was taken ill and was absent for two or three months. In 1915 the Asylum employed Dr. Stevens as Assistant Medical Officer.

During the war doctors were in short supply as the younger men were called to the front. In 1914 Dr. Gage joined the Royal Navy. During this time, Dr. Caldecott was virtually alone and the work was hard. His only recreation was cricket, which he loved. From 1917 onwards Dr. Bowes, who had himself been a Medical Superintendent of an institution, assisted him.

Dr. Caldecott was very popular. He knew every patient and their history. Staff reported that he knew everything that went on in the Asylum. He was very strict but everyone took their work seriously and did the best they could. He appreciated the effort. He would not tolerate drunkenness and persistent lateness but he also knew when to turn a blind eye according to one of the attendants, Percy Robinson.

There was a lack of teaching aids for the nursing staff and no study time. Dr. Caldecott would give lectures in the evening and allow the trainee nurses to bandage him. In 1923 Dr. Caldecott fell ill again and by August Dr. Dunscombe was deputising for him. He died shortly afterwards and the post of Medical Superintendent fell vacant.

The post was advertised, the following text appearing in the newspapers:

Royal Earlswood Institution
FOR MENTAL DEFECTIVES.
(Registered under the Mental Deficiency Act 1913)

The Board of Management invite applications for the post of MEDICAL SUPERINTENDENT from duly qualified and registered medical practitioners, under 40 years of age.
Salary £800 per annum, with furnished house in the main building, lighting and heating, laundry, and vegetables.

Applications, giving full particulars of qualifications and past experience, to be sent to the Secretary, at the London Offices, 14-16 Ludgate Hill, E.C.4, with copies of not more than four recent testimonials, marked "Medical Superintendent" and to be delivered on or before the 1st August.

14th July, 1923   H. HOWARD, Secretary.

Dr. Stephen Langton applied. He had trained at Middlesex Hospital and qualified MRCS and LRCP in 1911, after which he worked at the hospital for six months. From November 1911 until April 1913 he worked as the sixth Assistant Medical Officer at Claybury, London County Council Asylum. Meanwhile he studied and sat his MBBS examination at London University. He joined the Indian Medical Service in the summer of 1913 but due to the rigors of the climate he returned to Britain in March 1915. He then took a post as second Medical Officer at Berry Wood Asylum, with Northamptonshire County Council, for a few months.

In July 1915 Langton moved to Dorset where he had a private panel practice and was also surgeon for the Admiralty. In addition, he provided medical services for the Coast Guard Station Naval Base and Naval Sick Quarters. This involved responsibility for over 800 men. He must have been full of energy and not afraid of hard work as he was also in charge of the Municipal Isolation Hospital. With the severe shortage of doctors during the First World War, in 1917 he also became medical officer to the Royal Navy Air Service Aerodrome at Lipton, Medical Officer to the Royal Navy Cordite Factory at Wareham and the RAF Depot Sandbank.

Following the end of the war Langton moved north and became the deputy Medical Superintendent and deputy Mental Deficiency Officer at York City Mental Hospital. He provided a specialist service in neurology and carried out lumber punctures and other surgical procedures. He remained at York until his successful application for the position of Medical Superintendent and Resident Physician at Earlswood.

Dr. Langton took a very active interest in the running of the Institution. He was concerned with cost efficiency. His mother lived in the hospital and had quite an influence over him. A large collection of memoranda survives in which he specifies rules, regulations and the way in which the day-to day functioning of the Asylum should occur. There are thirty-six for 1935 alone. Topics included such diverse issues as:

> The securing of rooms.
> The cleaning of the dining room floor with
> turpentine rather than water.
> The way the stairs should be cleaned.
> The clothing of the clients.
> Employment regulations.
> The use of ladders.
> Methods of serving in the dining room.
> Lost property.
> Emptying of dustbins.
> The taking of temperatures.
> The serving of jam.
> The amount and type of polish to be used on
> different surfaces etc.

In 1938 Stephen Langton resigned due to ill health. At this time there was concern about the salary being paid to the Medical Officers of the hospital. The Medical Superintendent was paid £800 plus accommodation, the deputy Superintendent £350-£500 and the junior Medical Officer only £250-£350, £100 below the normal rate for the job. Dr. Langton was replaced by the deputy Superintendent, Dr. Henry Robb Ferguson. Dr. Ferguson had qualified in Glasgow in 1927. He spent a year at Bethlem Royal Hospital before joining Royal Earlswood in 1928. He remained as Physician Superintendent until his retirement in 1964. Throughout this time he was resident in quarters within the Hospital, available day and night and reputedly he knew every resident by name. Relieved of his responsibilities he did not enjoy a long retirement dying early in 1966.

By the 1960s the hospital had, in addition to the full time medical staff, a number of visiting doctors including an ophthalmologist, Dr. Curtis, a general practitioner, Dr. Johnson, and two anaesthetists, Dr. Gibbons and Dr. Law. There were also three visiting dental officers, Mr. Keith, Mr. Cramp and Mr. Scully.

In September 1972 Dr. Anderson, the last Physician Superintendent, retired and the management of services was put into the hands of a senior officers' Executive Committee, with power to act on all day-to-day issues. A team approach developed involving physicians, nurses, psychologists, occupational therapists and all professional staff in the running of the increasingly complex organisation. The physical care of the residents was taken over by a team of general practitioners from the first of November 1973. Cricket remained a popular recreation for the medical staff of Earlswood, and they continued to do well. In 1976 the District

Consultants challenged Royal Earlswood and were all out for 103, Earlswood reached 103 for 3 wickets.

By 1979 there were nine medical staff to provide medical services across the three hospitals, Earlswood, Forest and Farmfield.

1865-70	**Dr. George Shuttleworth**
1868-?76	**Dr. White**
?1876-?	**Dr. Spence**
1904-10	**Dr. Pearce**
1904	**Dr. Whittingham**
1906	**Dr. Thomson**
?	**Dr. Pierce, Dr. Rankin**
1911	**Dr. Nelson - Assistant Medical Officer**
1912-14	**Dr. Gage**
1915	**Dr. Stevens**
1917	**Dr. Bowes**
1923	**Dr. Dunscombe-(Acting Medical Superintendent Aug-Sept 1938)**
1928	**Dr. Ferguson, deputy medical superintendent from 1937-8**
1929	**Dr. Donald Hood CNO MD FRCP – Consulting physician to the Institution**
1937-39	**Dr. Fossard, Dr. Lynch**
1940	**Dr. Sim**
1940-43	**Dr. Cunningham**
1941-43	**Dr. Ruff**
1942-43	**Dr. L A B Moore**
1946-47	**Dr. Ritchie**
1950-64	**Dr. Anderson – joined as a second consultant. In 1964 took over as Medical Superintendent.**
1951-54	**Dr. Mansell**
1951-66	**Dr. McLeod**
1952-66	**Dr. Gurney-Smith**
1954-59	**Dr. G J F Fryer**
1958	**Dr. Grant M.B., Ch.B., D.P.M – Asst. psychiatrist and senior hospital medical officer.**
1959-76	**Dr. Roger Mirrey M.B., B.S., D.P.M.– reached level of deputy medical superintendent and Consultant psychiatrist. Retired March 1976.**
1965	**Dr. . Banerjee**
1972	**Dr. Barron**
1973	**Dr. Peard – paediatrician**
1974	**Dr. Gibson – Consultant psychiatrist**
1976-2004	**Dr. Kio Vejdani – Consultant psychiatrist**

Other Medical Staff mentioned in documents with date of mention.

Annual Festivals

The Festival Dinners held annually by the Charity were a means of publicising the work of the Asylum and raising money with which to continue that work. They provided an opportunity to build up a list of regular subscribers. The plan to construct a purpose-built Asylum at Earlswood was announced at the dinner in 1850 and the building fund was launched. The

Royal Family provided considerable support in this as in many other ways. In 1871 the Prince of Wales presided at the dinner and H.R.H. Duke of Cambridge took the chair on two occasions. At the request of Dr. Conolly, Charles Dickens consented to become a steward at the dinner in 1851.

Date		President (and subscription)	Total Contributions.
1856	March 27th	The Lord Mayor	
1857	March 30th	Lord Monteagle	
1858	March 31st	Duke of Wellington	
1859	April 12th	Lord Mayor, Sir George Carroll	
1860	March 9th	H.R.H. The Duke of Cambridge	
1861	February 12th	Lord Stanley, Earl of Derby	
1862	March 4th	Lord Mayor, Alderman Cubitt	
1863	March 4th	Alderman Abbiss, in absence of Lord Calthorpe	£1.980.00
1864	March 17th	Charles Buxton, Esq. M.P. (50guineas)	£2,500.00
1865	March 22nd	Sir Fraser H. Goldsmid, M.P. (100guineas)	£2,000.00
1866	February 28th	Lord Dufferin K.C.B.	£2,300.00
1867	March 25th	Lord Mayor, Alderman Gabriel.	£5,000.00
1868	March 27th	Sir T. Fowell Buxton.	
1869	March 11th	Sir John Lubbock.	
1870	February 23rd	J.D. Allcroft, Esq.	
1871	May 17th	H.R.H. Prince of Wales.	
1872	April 30th	Colonel R. Lloyd Lindsay.	
1873	March 6th	Lord Mayor, Sir S.H. Waterlow.	
1874	April 22nd	The Rt. Hon. S. Cave, M.P.	£2,400.00
1875	April 18th	Lord Mayor, Alderman Stone.	£2,294.00
1876	March 15th	The Earl of Shaftsbury	£2,172.00
1877	March 9th	Francis Peek, Esq. (£50)	£3,613.00
1878	May 3rd	Sir T. Chambers, M.P.	£1,594.00
1879	May 20th	Baron Henry de Worms.	£2,900.00
1880	April 22nd	The Earl of Rosebery.	£2,259.00
1881	March 22nd	J.J. Colman, Esq. M.P.	
1882	April 21st	Mr. Alderman Fowler, M.P.	£2,631.00
1883	March 7th	The Rt. Hon. G.J. Goshen, M.P.	£1,000.00
1884	March 24th	Richard K. Causton, Esq. M.P.	
1885	March 3rd	Lord Herschell.	
1886	April 8th	Sir Trevor Lawrence, M.P.	
1887	March 22nd	H.R.H. The Duke of Cambridge.	
1888	April 13th	Sir J. Whittaker Ellis, Bart. M.P.	
1889	March 13th	J.C. Parkinson, Esq. J.P., D.L.	
1890	March 12th	Alfred L. Cohen, Esq. (100 guineas)	£5,847.98
1891	May 20th	Sir J. Blundell Maple (100guineas)	£4,000.00
1892	May 3rd	Alderman George Faudell Phillips (100guineas)	£2,850.36
1893	June 28th	Alderman I. Voce Moore. (20guineas)	£1,922.35
1894	March 15th	H.L.W. Hawson, Esq. M.P. (100guineas)	£2,086.00
1895	April 9th	Alderman Sir Joseph Dimsdale, (50guineas)	£2,075.01
1896	May 13th	Alderman Marens Samuel (100guineas)	£3,317.55
1898	May 20th	The Duke of Leeds (60guineas)	£2,125.38
1899	May 9th	Lord Chief Justice, Lord Russell of Killowen (£5)	£3,108.18
1901	March 14th	Rt. Hon. Lord Battersea (50guineas)	£2,434.37
1902	June 18th	E.C.P. Hull, Esq. J.P. (100guineas)	£2,427.43
1903	March 31st	Jeremiah Colman, Esq. D.L., J.P. (£500)	£2,936.43
1904	April 19th	Rt. Hon. Lord Rothschild, (500guineas)	£4,321.60
1906	June 18th	Rt. Hon. Lord Mayor, Alderman W. Vaughan Morgan (20guineas)	£4,134.70
1907	May 9th	Hon. Alban Gibbs, M.A. (50guineas)	£2,924.30
1908	May 20th	Rt. Hon. Lord Collins (20guineas)	£1,696.49
1909	May 11th	Sir Felix Schuster, Bart. (70guineas)	£3,160.92
1910	July 15th	Colonel R.H. Rawson, M.P. (10guineas)	£1,715.52
1911	May 31st	William Hartmann, Esq. J. P. (£200)	£2,150.52
1912	May 23rd	Almeric Paget, Esq. M.P. (50guineas)	£2,441.25
1913	April 23rd	Sir Frederick J. Mirrielees K.C.M.G. (150guineas)	£2,073.05
1914	June 3rd	E.C.P. Hull, Esq. J.P. (100guineas)	£2,237.34
		THE GREAT WAR	
1922	May 1st	Sir Ralph C. Forster, Bart. D.L., J.P. (£500)	£3,253.85
1923	Dec 11th	Major General, The Earl of Athlone, G.C.B.,G.C.V.O.,G.C.M.G., D.S.O.	£2,230.00

Record of the Annual Festivals.

In 1863 the dinner was held at the London Tavern in Bishopsgate, London. A founding member of the Charity, Alderman Abbiss, presided. Mrs. Plumbe and Charles Reed, the son of the recently deceased founder Andrew Reed, were amongst the 150 who attended. The following words were sung at the Festival Dinner:

> "Use him fairly, he will prove
> How the simple heart can love;
> He will spring with infant glee
> To the form he likes to see.
> Gentle speech, or kindness done,
> Truly binds the witless one."

In 1864 the Member of Parliament for Maidstone, Charles Buxton, was in the chair. There were 200 in attendance and contributions of nearly £2,500 were announced on the night. There

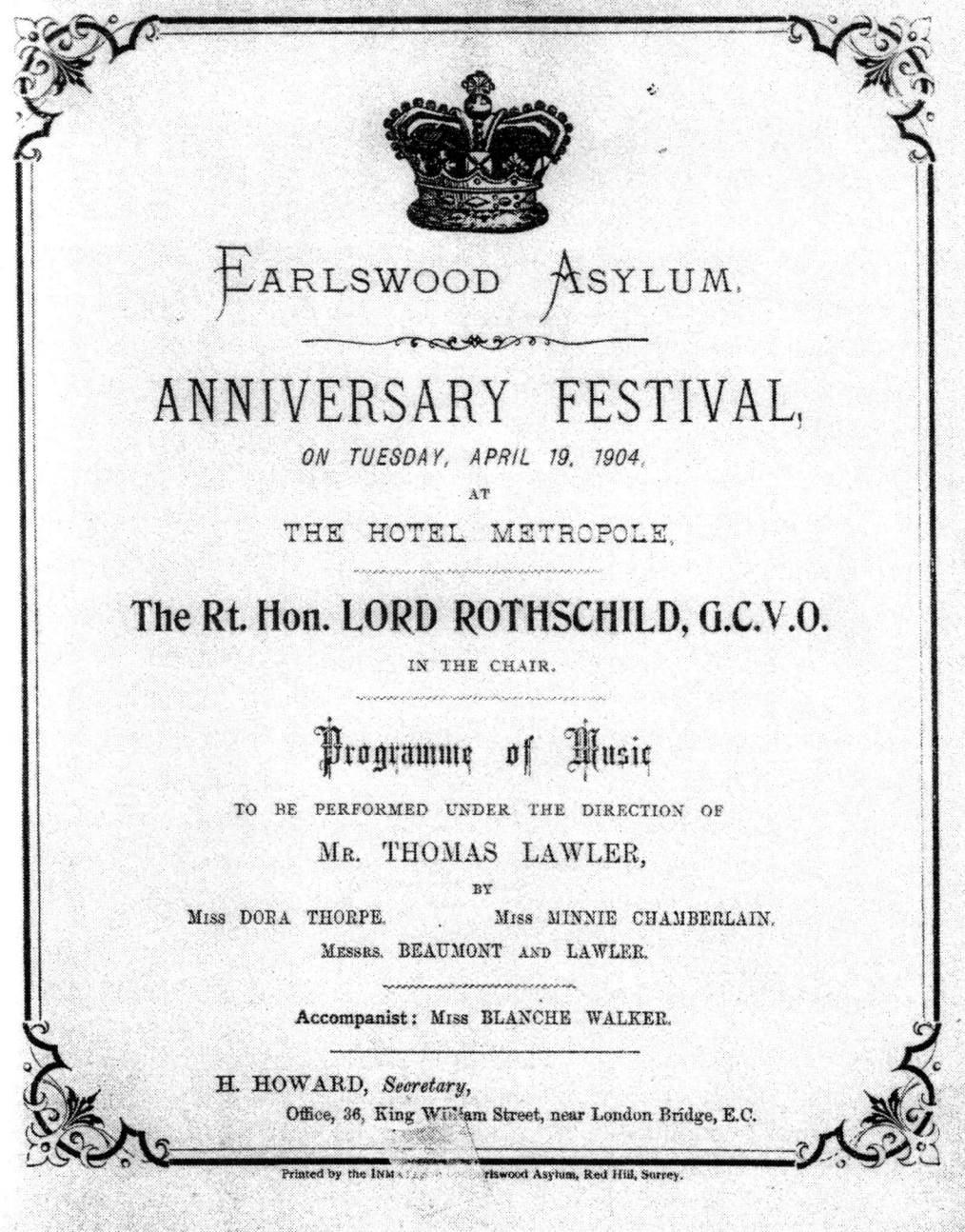

was a single anonymous donation of £525. The dinner continued to be held at the London Tavern in 1865 and 1866 with 160 attending on each occasion. In 1867 there were 200 paying guests, the Lord Mayor of London presided. The evening initially raised £4,900 but the chair challenged nineteen guests to pledge £5 each if he would do the same. The result was one of the highest totals recorded at a Festival Dinner.

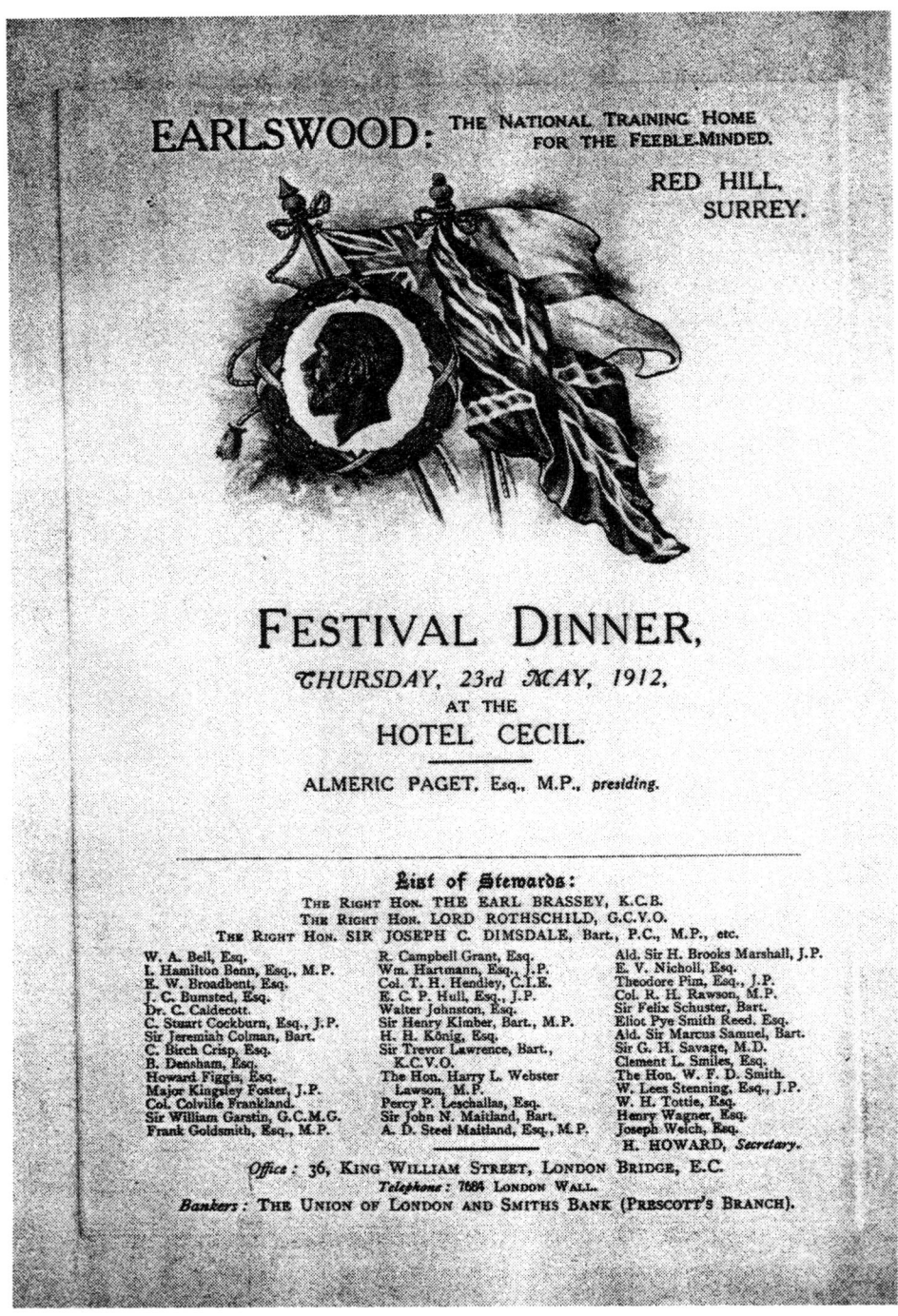

In 1875 the dinner was once again presided over by a Lord Mayor of London. The need for an infirmary was highlighted and a special appeal was made. The cost would be £1,800. Until 1876 the Festival Dinner continued to be held at The London Tavern. In 1877 the venue moved to the Albion Tavern, Aldersgate Street. There were 120 present including the Director of the Bank of England and several of his staff. The diners heard of a previous inmate, who now worked as a nurse in a family, another employed as a shoemaker and a third who worked as an elementary teacher. In 1879 the evening raised £2,900 including a single anonymous gift of

£500. The following year the 120 paying guests were given the welcome news that the Charity had succeeded in clearing its debts although further funds were still required for the construction of the infirmary.

Those attending the dinner in 1882 were encouraged to contribute further to the Charity as it was announced that 2041 pupils had passed through the Asylum since its establishment. The Institution accommodated 563 at the time. Given sufficient funds a further 200 needy souls could benefit from the training that Earlswood had to offer. In Sydney, Australia a similar hospital was being built at a cost of £200,000.

On the 18th of June 1906 the Annual Festival Dinner was presided over by the Lord Mayor, Alderman W. Vaughan Morgan at the Haberdashers Hall in London. Approximately one hundred guests attended. In 1907 the dinner provided the opportunity to launch a special appeal for the £25,000 building fund for the rebuilding of the east wing of the Asylum, made necessary by the deficiencies in the original construction of Earlswood. Mr. Hull, the Chairman of the Board, donated £500.

The Festival Dinners provided an opportunity to report on the progress being made by some of the residents at Earlswood. In 1909 the guests were told of a man whose mind had improved so significantly that he had started his own cabinet-making business, using skills acquired and perfected at the Asylum. Most inmates were usefully employed on profitable work.

In 1910 the dinner had to be postponed from June the 10th until the 15th of July as a result of the death of Edward VII. The subscriptions received were reduced as people felt the pinch of new taxation that had been introduced in the country. It was suggested that Earlswood should change its name as the term 'asylum' made many people think of the mentally ill. 'Home' or 'institution' was proposed as an alternative. The Festival Dinners were suspended in 1915 as a result of the First World War. They did not resume until 1922.

Pullen

One resident of Earlswood was famous during his lifetime. James Henry Pullen demonstrated extraordinary talents that excited interest from the media. The officers of the Charity, always conscious of the need to raise public awareness if funds were to follow, were happy that the Asylum should exploit this for maximum benefit.

Pullen was born in London, probably Dalston, on the second of August 1835. His parents were first cousins, which may explain the fact that Pullen and two of his brothers suffered from disabilities leading to their admission to the Asylum. James was one of thirteen children, six of whom died in infancy and four in later childhood. He had difficulty hearing and was reputedly born without a roof to his mouth. He began to talk at seven years of age, speaking with a lisp and using disjointed words. He is believed to have had a communication disorder making the construction of sentences difficult if not impossible. No school would accept him and he apparently spent his early years drawing or carving ships.

It took two years for sufficient votes to be accumulated for his application to be successful. He was admitted to Essex Hall in May 1850 and was amongst the first to transfer to Earlswood when it opened in 1855. On admission he was well grown being over five foot, seven inches tall and nearly ten stones. He was able to care for himself. In the Annual Report of 1853 the following description certainly refers to Pullen:

> "**Case 9. – J.P., a boy, aged seventeen years. Admitted, *May*, 1850. He could neither read nor write; had a slight idea of drawing; was very unsociable, passionate, and self-willed, and was nearly deaf and dumb. *April*, 1853. He can read a little, can write and draw well, is very playful and attentive to orders, has greatly improved in speaking and hearing, and is an excellent mechanic.**"

Pullen had many talents including his ability to draw and paint, to carve, to design and construct objects in wood. He was a competent draughtsman and mechanic. He was also trained in photography. A number of his projects survive and continue to astound those who view them with their ingenuity and beauty. He constructed lockless boxes that only he could open and 'puzzles of many pieces' that he sold for sixpence (2.5p). Pullen in his youth was described as a master fencer.

Pullen had his own workshop at the hospital that became know as Pullen's room. He made various magnifiers and reflectors to help with his fine carving. In the room there were drawings that explained his life. There were sketches of him in the various workshops crying because he could not get on, in the brush making shop crying because he did not like the work and then him in carpentry shop, smiling as he had found his niche.

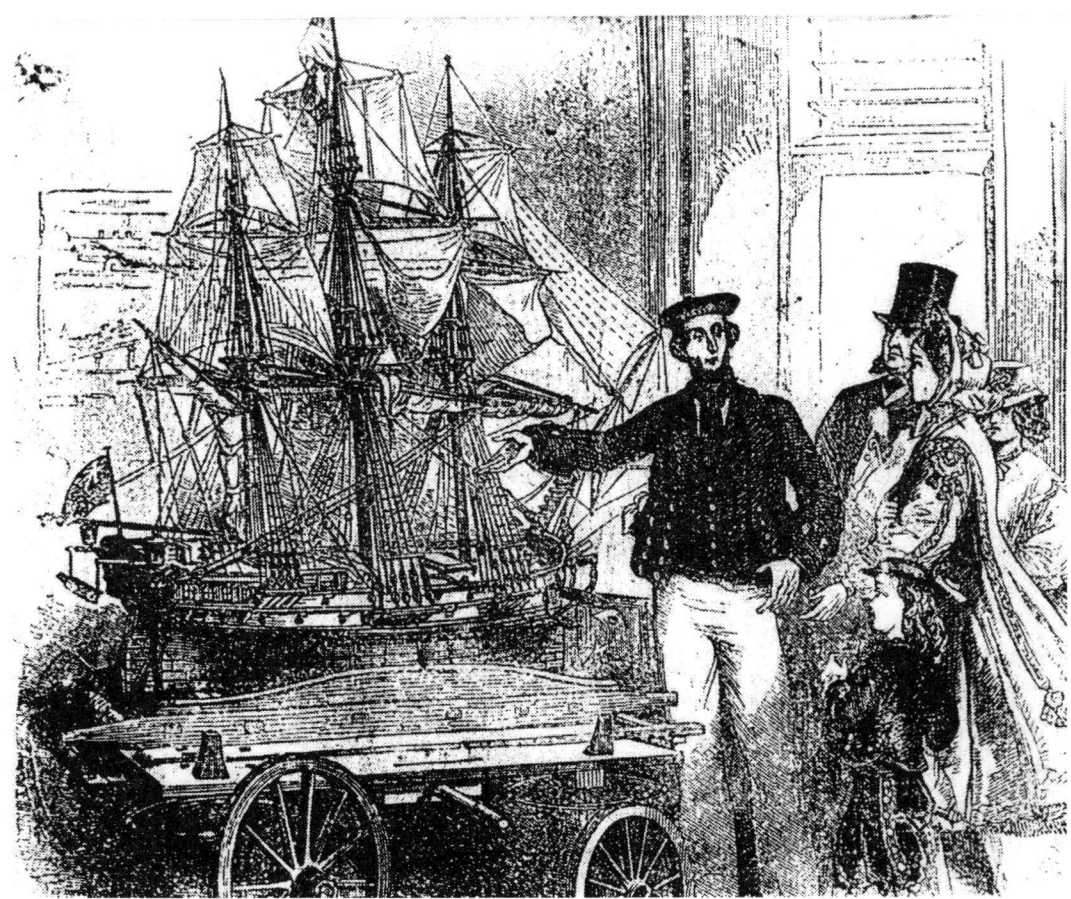

Pullen exhibiting the 'H.M.S Alexandra'.

'The Sheffield Times' of the 11th November 1862 recorded the completion by Pullen of his Man'o'war, a project that had taken him seven years to complete. A model of a ship of the line,

Pullen had copied the design from a picture on a four-penny handkerchief. Small copper plates protected its hull, all hand riveted. It contained 5,585 copper rivets and was complete with cargo in the hold. The rigging contained 200 individual pulley blocks. The model was exhibited at the International Exhibition in 1862 and was displayed at the summer fete in 1863. Alderman Abbiss named her the H.M.S. Alexandra after H.R.H Princess of Wales. The band played Rule Britannia. She was later exhibited in the front hall of Earlswood.

Pullen had visited several dockyards where the workings of the ships were explained to him. He also gained much from the ex-sailors that made up a proportion of the male attendants at Earlswood. One of Pullen's greatest works is his model of the Great Eastern. In 1861 he was given a shilling model of the Great Eastern for his Christmas present. Pullen was taken to the Great Exhibition in 1862. He saw the Great Eastern and spent an hour or two studying and sketching. On his return he could not settle until he had drawn the ship and begun to work out how to construct a life-like replica.

Pullen's 'modus operandi' seems to have been to repeatedly draw his design, from every angle, until he was sure of how it should look. The Great Eastern took three years and three months to complete. Before starting work on the boat itself he constructed a cradle on which to create his masterpiece. The boat was held together with one and a quarter million tiny wooden pins, each manufactured by Pullen on a special instrument that he had designed and built himself. The model was ten foot long and nearly nineteen inches wide. The ship was complete with furnished cabins inside that could be viewed by raising the deck using a system of pulleys. The model contained staterooms for only two classes, Royalty and the poor, Pullen knew of none between.

He also constructed a gun carriage to transport his creation, together with a launcher. The model was eventually launched on the Earlswood lakes at the Summer Festival. It apparently sank as Pullen had failed to understand the principles of buoyancy. However, he did successfully modify the model. The boat was launched sideways, as was its namesake on the Thames. The great paddle steamer, originally called the Leviathan, was built on the Isle of Dogs and like the model that bore its name the launch did not go according to plan. Originally scheduled for November 3rd 1857, the ship failed to move and was not successfully floated for over a year.

The Great Eastern was exhibited at the International Fisheries Exhibition in 1883 and was then on display in the Charity's London Office at 36 King William Street. The Great Eastern was subsequently on display every year at the Earlswood Summer Festival.

Following the construction of the Great Eastern, records indicate that in 1866 Pullen was working on a large state barge, painted in the colours of the rainbow. Dr. Down arranged for his work to be exhibited at the international exhibition in Paris and it won a bronze medal. Subsequently, he made a Chinese junk.

One of his most interesting constructions was a 'fantasy' boat. Pullen described it as a globe, representing the world, on a galley ship powered by oars. At the prow was a carved ivory figure, a representation of 'Satan subdued' and the stern held ivory angels, a sun and a moon. Pullen reputedly designed and built the ship as a vessel fit to transport Queen Victoria up the Thames. Inside the smooth maple wood dome, only about 25 centimetres across, are visible chairs and a table, complete with small pads of paper, a sceptre, orb and a red dispatches box.

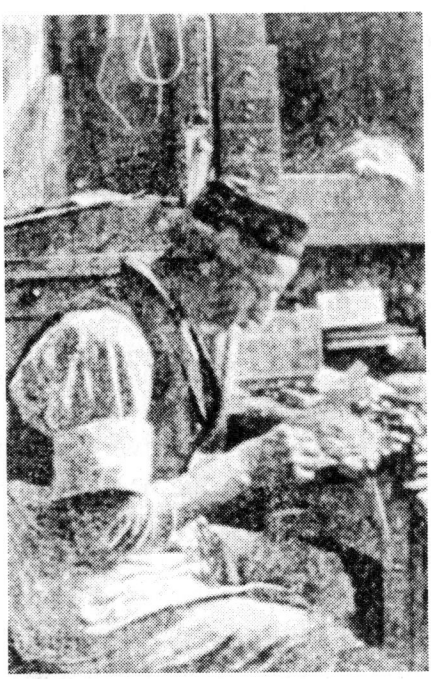

James Henry Pullen at work

Another of his unusual projects was an ivory landscape brooch. A piece of tortoiseshell at the back, with a judicious arrangement of golden and dark blotches, made it a transparency. When held up to the light, on one side it was a sunny scene, whilst on the other it was dark with a full moon.

Pullen drew many pictures including images of Sebastopol from his imagination. He constructed a huge kite for the children at Earlswood. He was the only resident to play in the Asylum band. He played the drums.

Also in the workshop, was Pullen's 'Giant', a large figure approximately thirteen feet tall, constructed of wood, fabric and paint, and apparently modelled on the figure of a Russian hussar. Pullen regarded it as his protecting deity. The eyes, made of canvas with bristles as lashes, could be opened and closed. The arms were operated by levers inside the body, which was large enough to accommodate a small man. A megaphone, in the shape of a plume on the front of the hat, allowed the voice to be projected. The giant was brought out each year on the day of the summer fete and Pullen exhibited it with great pride. In addition to Pullen's room there was a second apartment in which his works were exhibited.

Both sides of the Hospital corridor were hung with Pullen's paintings and prints. It is reported that, in a fit of temper, he broke his leg and Dr. Down had to set it. Whilst he was immobilised he took up painting as a way of passing the time. Landseer, a famous artist of the time, sent him a number of engravings that he copied superbly.

Pullen came to the attention of the highest in the land. Following the ceremony for the opening of Earlswood the Prince Consort accepted, on behalf of the Queen, one of his Landseer copies and it was hung in her private apartments at Windsor. She sent him in return two guineas in pocket money. Edward, Prince of Wales, was so impressed by Pullen's work that he afterwards sent him two elephant tusks. Pullen carved ivory brooches and tiepins and incorporated ivory into a number of his models.

Pullen was employed for six months in 1881 building a library cabinet for a private patient. He had extraordinary freedom compared to the other residents of Earlswood. He alone was allowed to leave the Institution in the evening to sell items that he had made. He would go out at 6.30pm with his sale goods in a brown paper bag. He would tour the public houses of the town, starting first with the New Inn before moving on to the Greyhound and the Warwick. He would buy himself a drink, usually scotch, and sell a brooch or tiepin for 2s 6d (12.5p) or 3s 6d (17.5p). He followed this pattern for a number of years returning by the deadline of 10pm. However, Mr. Wells, a schoolmaster, recorded that one night he was brought home the worst for drink and after curfew. Dr. Caldicott said that he was not to go out again until further notice and must not drink. Pullen became teetotal from that time on. He was allowed to resume his outings three months later.

Pullen was a complex character. He worked alone and was jealous of assistance. Nobody was allowed to touch his models. After his midday meal he would go to his workshop. He would climb a rope ladder to a platform that he had constructed near the top windows where the light was better. He would pull the ladder up behind him and have a sleep. Pullen would balance books on top of the door so that they would drop on the head of anyone entering.

Pullen was always well dressed. He had tight fitting kid gloves and a gold watch. He generally wore a naval uniform. The story of how Pullen acquired this may be of some interest. Pullen, on one of his outings, apparently met and believed himself in love with a local girl. He declared his intention to leave the Institution, which he was at liberty to do. However, he was an important generator of funds and the Board were unwilling to lose him. Pullen was summoned to the Boardroom and offered a naval uniform and the title of Admiral of the Fleet of Earlswood if he would agree to remain in the Asylum. He reputedly thought about this for thirty seconds and chose the uniform. He never again mentioned the girl.

Pullen finally died on the 31st of May 1916 at the age of nearly 81. He had been in an Asylum for about 66 years, almost entirely at Earlswood. The cause of death was recorded as senility and cardiac syncope. Dr. F Sano carried out a post mortem study of Pullen's brain. He published a report in the Journal of Mental Science in July 1918.

> **"The brain was small; its frontal and temporal lobes are badly developed: there is a lack of complexity in the convolutional patterns of these lobes and this is obviously marked in the speech centre. His deaf mutism was more central than peripheral in origin. The parietal lobes were not so bad, the occipital lobes were good, the corpus callosum was remarkable and he was bound to have special capacity in the visual sphere of his mental existence."**

The evidence suggests that Pullen's diagnosis was 'Isolation Ament', i.e. a person whose brain failed to develop fully owing to lack of stimulation, several avenues having been blocked, namely his hearing and speech.

Pullen's younger brother William Arthur was admitted to Earlswood in 1862 at the age of eight. His admission papers gave the following as evidence of his disability: "His countenance and actions proclaim his unfortunate condition. Great difficulty in managing him – very noisy at times, a propensity to play with fire." The schoolmaster listed him in 1869 as a fulltime pupil of the school and amongst those who had made particular progress. In 1871 he was part time at school and the remaining time was spent in the carpenters shop. He was also artistic and was eventually trained as a lithographic printer. He left Earlswood and gained employment outside. However, he was readmitted for some reason in December 1889 and the supervisor of the print shop reported that he had lost none of his ability and could safely be left to undertake any

THE SILENT WORKER.

AN EPISODE OF THE ROYAL EARLSWOOD INSTITUTION.

BY MARGARET McMILLAN.

Author of "*Labour and Childhood.*"

THE people who cannot march with the army, the so-called failures, the unfit, are to be found everywhere. Some are striving hopelessly to keep pace with the efficient, some are being helped along somehow in the rear, some are trampled under foot, and some are in Homes and Refuges. They may repay looking at just as well as do jewels—or strange manuscripts.

In Earlswood every order of disqualified person is gathered. The Inmates, for one reason or another, cannot face life alone. Yet they are not destitute of capacity. Many are capable of good work, and are indefatigable and laborious. The workers who go on tirelessly and never care to stop are, strange to say, the most hopeless cases, whose brains work like a machine, and who apparently never reach the sources of a higher energy. A few work quite aimlessly. One old man has written nonsense for years.

Finally genius is to be found at Earlswood—shining out gloriously amid the wreckage of a great life.

Here, for example, is a wonderful room. It looks like a shop and studio combined. There are strange paintings (that reminded me of Goethe's early efforts displayed in the Goethe house at Frankfurt), and everywhere beautiful carving, lockless boxes that no one but the maker can open. On a low table near the fire is a box full of lovely ivory carved brooches.

Yes, this is genius—bold, solitary, beautiful. Working with a dreamy look on his pale face, passing his well-kept hands over every tool and over his material, ere he uses them, as if to take them into a strange secret, the man of genius lives here alone. Language is a tool which he can hardly be said to use. At the age of seven he began to speak. Now he will sometimes utter words in a husky whisper. They are for the most part unintelligible. Alone, far away he is from all, working, finding, inventing, dreaming.

" How beautiful the brooches are !"

Recalled by these words, he turned from his work, took the brooches out of their boxes, and showed the names of the flowers they represented written in Latin, and then, as a warmer wave of sympathy reached him, put down the trinkets suddenly, smiled, and prepared to show us some of the masterpieces of his life-long labours.

They are real masterpieces—not broken dreams.

Of course, one does not stumble continually at Earlswood on suggestions of human greatness. Very often, however, one stumbles on suggestions of human weakness that are so familiar, so common that one might very well imagine oneself outside.

In the large workshops, the bootmakers' room, the tailors', the printers', the carpenters', the smiths' shops, hundreds are busy all day long, but now as the afternoon light wanes the workers lay aside their tasks for a while. From the great music-room where the children and women are gathered a flood of melody pours forth like a stream, lights waken in the dim corridors and rooms, and rosy curtains hide the sadness of the waning autumn day. Earlswood is a home as well as a refuge. It is a school as well as a workshop. As one passes down the wet avenue, where the yellow foliage shines like two lines of light athwart the rain, one hopes that the number of its helpers will increase, and that no new calamity will touch its helpless Inmates or close the door on the many who long to enter and be at peace.

Buck & Wootton, Ltd., Printers, 126 Westminster Bridge Road, S.E.

aspect of work in the shop. He sadly died on the 2nd of October 1893 from a cancerous tumour of the upper jaw. He had been taken to a London Hospital and surgery performed in an attempt to remove the tumour. Unfortunately, the cancer returned. He was only 38 years old.

Annual Summer Entertainment Day.

This was the other name given to the Fete Day at Earlswood in the mid-nineteenth century. It was another important occasion for increasing public awareness and raising funds for the Asylum. As such it was generally well attended by the members of the Board. The importance of such a day for the finances of the Asylum can be seen by the reduction in income on years when the fete did not occur. In 1897, when the fete did not take place, life subscriptions and donations totalled £1,303 and £690 respectively. This compared poorly with the following year

---

EARLSWOOD ASYLUM.

FANCY FAIR & ANNUAL SUMMER FÊTE,

FOR THE AMUSEMENT OF THE INMATES,

THURSDAY, JUNE 20th, 1867.

TO COMMENCE AT ONE, P.M.

AMUSEMENTS ON THE LAWN.

Cricket; Croquet; Aunt Sally; Red, White, and Blue; Punch and Judy; Foot-Ball, &c.

3-30 P.M.

Racing and Jumping Matches, for Prizes, to be competed for by Boys engaged in the various branches of Industry.

5 P.M.

Tea of the Inmates on the Lawn.

6-15 P.M.

GLEES BY THE EARLSWOOD CHORAL UNION.

7 P.M.

ASCENT OF FIRE BALLOON.

7-30 P.M.

NEGRO MELODIES by the EARLSWOOD TROUPE.

To conclude at Eight p.m.

THROUGHOUT THE DAY THERE WILL BE

A SALE

OF USEFUL AND ORNAMENTAL ARTICLES

AT MODERATE PRICES.

The Band of the Coldstream Guards will be in attendance,

By the kind permission of Col. Ducket Carleton.

ADMISSION ONE SHILLING EACH PERSON,

Which will be returned in value from Articles in the Fancy Fair.

TICKETS can be obtained at Folthorp's Royal Library, Brighton; Messrs. Shuter, Reigate; Weller, Redhill; at the Asylum, Earlswood; and at the Office, 29, Poultry, London.
TICKETS for COLD COLLATION from One to Four, 1s. 6d., and for TEA and COFFEE, from Four to Seven, 1s.

LIGHT REFRESHMENTS AT A FIXED TARIFF.

The Brighton Company have kindly consented to grant RETURN TICKETS, First and Second Class, at Single Fares, viz.—3s. 8d. and 2s. 9d. between London and the NEW EARLSWOOD STATION, close to the Asylum, by the 12-10 p.m. and 2-10 p.m. Trains from London Bridge and Victoria; returning from Earlswood Station at 7-20 p.m. and 8-55 p.m.

Also between Brighton and Earlswood Station at 5s. 2d. & 3s. 10d., leaving Brighton at 11-30 a.m. and returning from Earlswood at 7-45 p.m. Tickets to be obtained ONLY at the Office, 29, Poultry, London, and at Folthorp's Royal Library, Brighton.

T. Weller, Printer, Redhill.

when the sums were swelled by the fete to £3,282 in the form of subscriptions and £1,168 in donations.

In 1863 the fete took place on Monday the 29th of June starting at one o'clock in the afternoon and finishing at eight in the evening. There were games and races with prizes for the winners. In early years these consisted of money ranging from a penny to a shilling (5p) for the residents

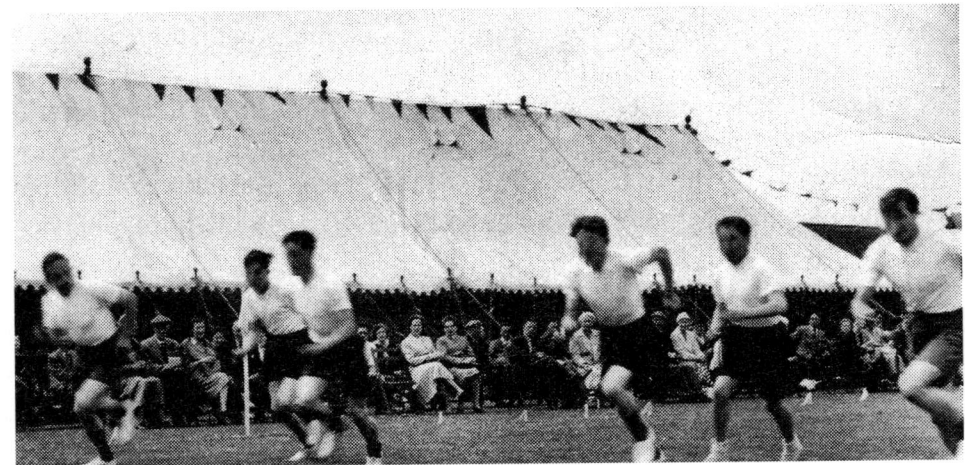

Sports day

and half a crown to ten shillings (12.5p to 50p) for the races involving the attendants. Later the rewards involved powder compacts for the women and cigarettes for the men – not suitable prizes according to modern ideas! Cricket and football matches provided plenty of opportunities for merriment amongst the spectators, especially with many of the Board members taking part. Croquet was a further entertainment available. There was a performance of glees by the singing class and the Earlswood Troupe sang Negro minstrel melodies. A shower of rain meant that tea had to be served in the main corridor of the Asylum, with tables set up along its length. Tea, cake and strawberries were all well received.

In 1866 the weather was kinder. Tea was served in the grounds, with the residents sitting on the grass in two large circles, one consisting of the men and boys and a separate one for the girls and women. It is recorded that the races that year occurred with Dr. Down striking a gong to set the runners off and Alderman Abbiss acting as the finishing post! The Asylum brass band generally played in the grounds and other bands of repute were often invited to provide entertainment for the residents and visiting guests. The Coldstream Guards Band attended on several occasions.

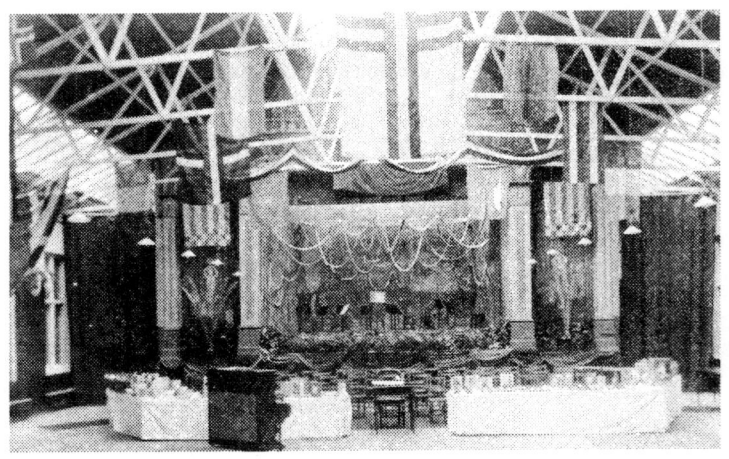

Entertainment Day

In 1867 the admission charge for the 'Summer fete and Fancy Fair' was one shilling (5p) with an extra charge of one shilling and sixpence (7.5p) for the cold collation. However, there were three tents of fancy goods from which items to the value of the admission charge could be chosen. The London and Brighton Railway Company offered return tickets for the price of a single to anyone who could present an admission ticket to the Fete. This was yet another example of the generosity regularly shown to the Asylum by the Company. It is recorded that 3000 visitors attended that year. A special train carried the passengers to the new station at Earlswood, open for the first time.

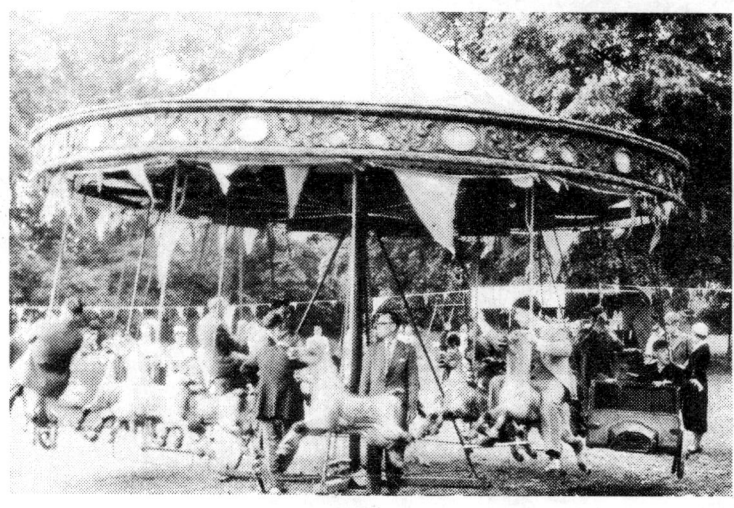

Summer fete day

Of particular interest each year was the ascent of the fire balloon. This did not always go without incident. In 1862 the balloon caught fire before the planned ascent could take place. The patients enjoyed this tremendously. The schoolmaster's journal contains the design for several of these balloons. In 1866 the balloon had a circumference of 37 feet, a length of just over twenty feet and was made up of 24 sections. It was fifteen foot nine inches tall when inflated. The design became grander every year. In 1867 the balloon was thirty feet high. The balloons were decorated with mottoes and sentiments appropriate for the era, wishes for the success of the Royal Family, the Nation and the Institution.

11.45	Pupils dine.	
12.30	Officers and servants dine.	
1.00	Pupils round the grounds Cricket, croquet, games	Balloon 15 feet high Wind S.W. very slight Lit up from front lawn,
3.00	Punch and Judy	Car and parachute
3.30	Racing	Parachute dropped just within grounds.
5.00	Tea on the lawn	
6.15	Choral Union	
7.00	Balloon	
7.30	Negro Melodies	

Figure 1.   **Timetable for the Annual Fete Day, 1866.**

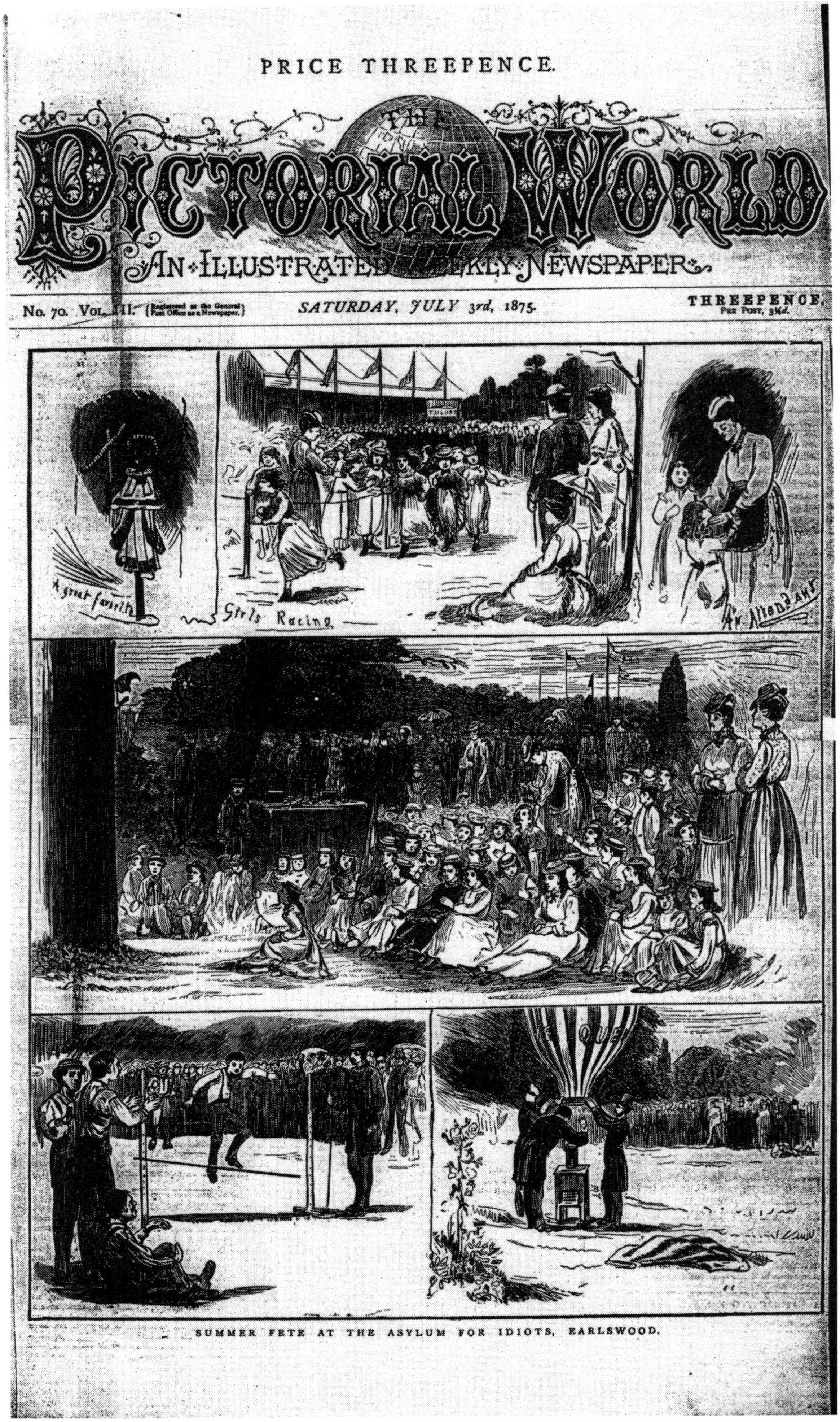

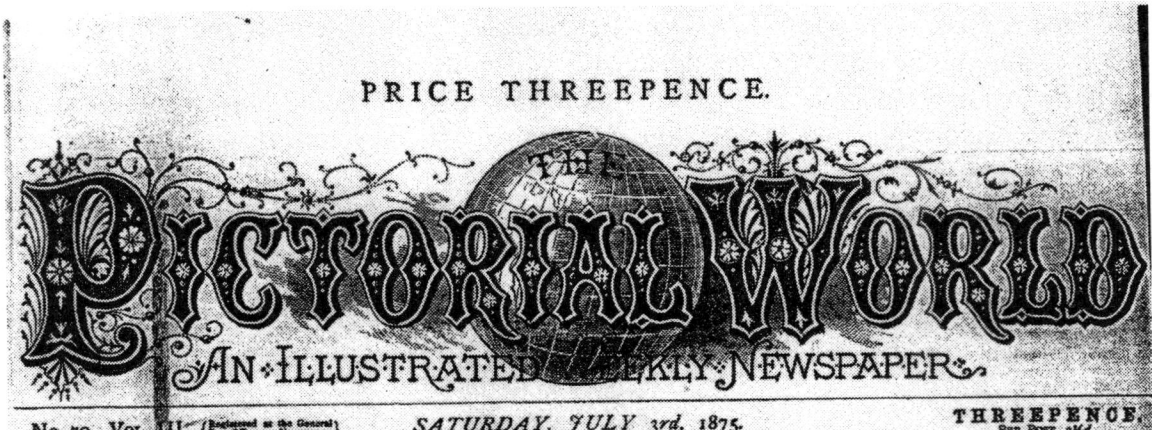

PRICE THREEPENCE.

THE PICTORIAL WORLD

AN·ILLUSTRATED·WEEKLY·NEWSPAPER·

No. 70. Vol. III. (Registered at the General Post Office as a Newspaper)   SATURDAY, JULY 3rd, 1875.   THREEPENCE. Per Post, 3½d.

A great forward — Girls Racing — Mr Allen & Ant

SUMMER FETE AT THE ASYLUM FOR IDIOTS, EARLSWOOD.

In 1874 there was a display in the dining room of handicrafts produced by the Asylum residents. The band of the Scots Fusilier Guards provided the music. It was recorded in the local paper that one inmate entertained the visitors with a troupe of performing mice; whilst several proudly displayed birds they had bred. Some sang songs to the great enjoyment of those attending, as well as themselves. Tea was taken in the covered playground and James Henry Pullen's proud work, the Great Eastern, was on display for the first time since its completion.

In 1876 in one tent a resident took photographs for sixpence, apparently they were of a very good standard. The Earlswood Negro Troop provided entertainment, nine attendants with their faces blackened and curly wigs. Pullen sold, for sixpence, wooden puzzles of many pieces that he had made. The residents' work was displayed in the dining room and tea was again served in the covered playground, the males on one side and the females on the other. The Great Eastern was again on display, together with a Chinese junk also made by Pullen. Balloons were a popular attraction with twenty taking part in a race.

In 1879 the fete commenced with a march, apprentices from the guilds carrying the banners of their trade. There were races and a Punch and Judy Show. This was followed by an ascent of 'grotesque' balloons. Tea was served in the main hall including cakes, nuts, oranges and sweets. The Asylum band played and the Earlswood Minstrels performed.

The Fete in 1883 was graced by the patronage of the Queen, the Prince and Princess of Wales and the Duke of Cambridge. The Presidents included two archbishops, the Duke of Wellington, the Earl of Chichester and a long list of Peers. Dinner was served to the Board and guests at 1pm. There were organ recitals during the day by James Halle of Clapham Congregational Church. The Coldstream Guards performed at 3pm and 6pm. One resident with a baton and a music stand beat time and seemed to believe he was in charge of the band. Other attractions included the hurdy-gurdy man and Ethiopian serenades. In 1891 the Band of the 14th Hussars provided the musical entertainment, supported by the Earlswood Asylum Military Band.

On the sixth of May 1927 the Surrey Mirror contained a preview of the Hospital Fete Day proposed to take place on the 27th of that month. Athletics and show jumping were planned. Each of the local boroughs was invited to nominate a runner for the 100 metres sprint. Other attractions included a pony competition, a performance by a concert party and dancing; the day was to end with fireworks. However, in the event, the fete had to be cancelled because of an outbreak of diphtheria at the Hospital.

The Earlswood Fete had to be suspended during the war years and it was June 1952 before it was reinstated. It then continued until the closure of the Hospital in 1997, subsequently transferring to Farmfield in Charlwood, location of three community-based assessment and treatment units. The fete generally took place in June, and later July, and the actual date was fixed by the availability of the large merry-go-round, a major attraction in later years.

Legislation

During the time of Edward II mentally abnormal citizens were recognised as falling into two groups, 'natural fools' and 'lunatics'. Care was limited to protecting their land and property and ensuring safe transfer to their heirs. Little was to change over the next 400 years. In 1815 'mental deficiency' was differentiated from 'mental disease', recognising the different

THE ROYAL EARLSWOOD INSTITUTION.

Notice to Patients.

The Hospital aims to provide all that is required for the care, treatment, and comfort of patients. They are invited, however, to make their wants and wishes known to the Sister or Charge Nurse of the Ward; or, if they prefer, direct to the Superintendent (verbally or in writing) or through one of the Medical or other Officers.

Official Visitors.

The Hospital is regularly visited by members of the Hospital Management Committee who see the patients and have the power of discharge. It is also visited from time to time by Commissioners of the Board of Control. All patients have the right to request a personal and private interview with a visiting Commissioner or with a member of the Hospital Management Committee when they visit the Hospital.

Letters.

No restrictions are normally placed on the receipt by patients of letters; but it is usually advisable that the contents of parcels should be examined.

Letters written by patients should be placed in the locked boxes provided for this purpose. They are collected at least once each day by a responsible Official.

Every patient has the right to have any letter sent unopened to :—

(a) the Management Committee of the Hospital or any member of the Committee;

(b) the Board of Control or any one of the Commissioners of the Board (32, Rutland Gate, Knightsbridge, London, S.W.7.);

(c) the Lord Chancellor (House of Lords, London, S.W.1.);

(d) the Minister of Health (Whitehall, London, S.W.1.);

(e) any Judge in Lunacy (Royal Courts of Justice, Strand, London, W.C.2.);

(f) the Chancery Visitors or any Chancery Visitor (Royal Courts of Justice, Strand, London, W.C.2);

(g) the person who signed the order for the patient's reception into the hospital;

(h) if a patient is resident under an order made on petition, the person on whose petition the order was made.

Apart from these letters, other letters before being posted may be examined by a Medical Officer or other responsible Official. When there is a doubt as to the propriety of their dispatch, the decision is a matter for the discretion of the Superintendent.

pathology and the need for a different management approach. However, when Earlswood was first founded there was no legal provision for those with a learning disability and they tended to be considered under the regulations laid down for the care of those with a mental illness.

Two Lunatics Acts passed in 1828 had required all local authorities to provide an asylum for the care and containment of 'Lunatics'. Often, those with a learning disability were accommodated in the same asylums. It was not until nearly 60 years later that the 'Permissive Idiots Act of 1886' allowed separate provision to be made for those with a learning disability and few local authorities chose to establish such institutions. Indeed, although the act specifically stated that the terms idiot and imbecile were not synonymous with 'lunatic', the 'Lunacy Act' of 1890 treated them as such.

Since the Earlswood Asylum was the first institution of its kind there was some doubt about its legal status. The 'Commissioners in Lunacy' claimed power of control and for many years the Asylum was subject to regular inspections by the Commissioners. The Asylum had to be registered as a Hospital and had to comply with all pertinent regulations. The Asylum was required to appoint a Resident Medical Superintendent as soon as possible. In the early days the Asylum fell foul of the regulations relating to the keeping of records and the transmission of copies to the Commissioners. This, amongst other factors, cost the first Medical Superintendent his position.

In 1870 the Metropolitan Asylum Board opened two Asylums for the learning disabled from London, at Leavesden for those in the north and Caterham for those in the south of the capital. It was suggested that all areas of the country should build an Asylum. Paid for by rates and public funds, each would house approximately 2000 adults and include a school for up to 500 children.

In 1881 the Government published a report that showed that there were 29,452 cases of learning disability in the country and only 3% were correctly accommodated, the remainder being in workhouses, prisons or lunatic asylums. The Elementary Education Act was passed in 1899, empowering all education authorities to set up classes or separate schools for children with a learning disability. The Defective and Epileptic Children (Education) Act, in the same year, permitted but did not compel the education of learning disabled children. By 1904 there were 9,000 children in special placements, over half of them in London. Earlswood was unusual for its long history of education provision in the provinces.

Also in 1904 a 'Royal Commission on the Care and Control of the Feeble-minded' was asked to report on the national situation. It took four years to consider all the evidence. It recognised a lack of provision for the welfare of the disabled, now known to number 60,000 in England and Wales.

> **"Of the gravity of the present state of things there is no doubt.......there are a number of mentally defective persons whose training is neglected, over whom no sufficient control is exercised and whose wayward and irresponsible lives are productive of crime and misery, of much injury and mischief to themselves and others."**

Legislation was slow to follow due to concern over the freedom of the individual. The legislation that did eventually result, the Mental Deficiency Act of 1913, enabled County and County Borough Councils to provide learning disability institutions. However, only £150,000 was provided from central Government, leaving Local Authorities to find a similar sum. This represented a halfpenny on the rates. Even so, the Chairman at the Annual Dinner on the 24th of April 1913 argued that the funding proposed in the new Government measures would be sufficient for only 10% of those identified by the Commission as being in need. Earlswood itself did not benefit from any of the funding that was directed at new institutions. The wisdom of this was questioned as established Asylums had the experience and it was argued that they should participate fully in the planned program.

From the first of April 1914 the Earlswood Asylum was certified under the Mental Deficiency Act. The act gave asylums the power of detention or 'certification' for a period of one year, renewable for five yearly periods. At the same time the name of the Asylum changed from 'The Earlswood Asylum for the Feeble-minded' to the Royal Earlswood Institution for Mental Defectives'. The act defined four classes of learning disability, idiots, imbeciles, and feeble-minded and moral defectives. The first three categories defined groups of rising intelligence, the idiot being the lowest. The last group consisted of persons with learning disability who, from their earliest days, demonstrated 'strong vicious or criminal propensities'. The terminology introduced by the act allowed the nature of disability to be described objectively and with some accuracy for the first time. This also helped in the development of social and medical research.

The act set up a central Board of Control and required local authorities to set up mental deficiency committees. They had responsibility for inspecting the hospitals at least twice yearly, for ensuring that all documentation and records were properly kept, for providing an annual report to Parliament and for overseeing the use of mechanical restraint and seclusion. The committees were also responsible for ensuring appropriate provision in each locality. From 1913 special schools were provided for 'feeble-minded' children eligible for certification under the Mental Deficiency Act or education acts

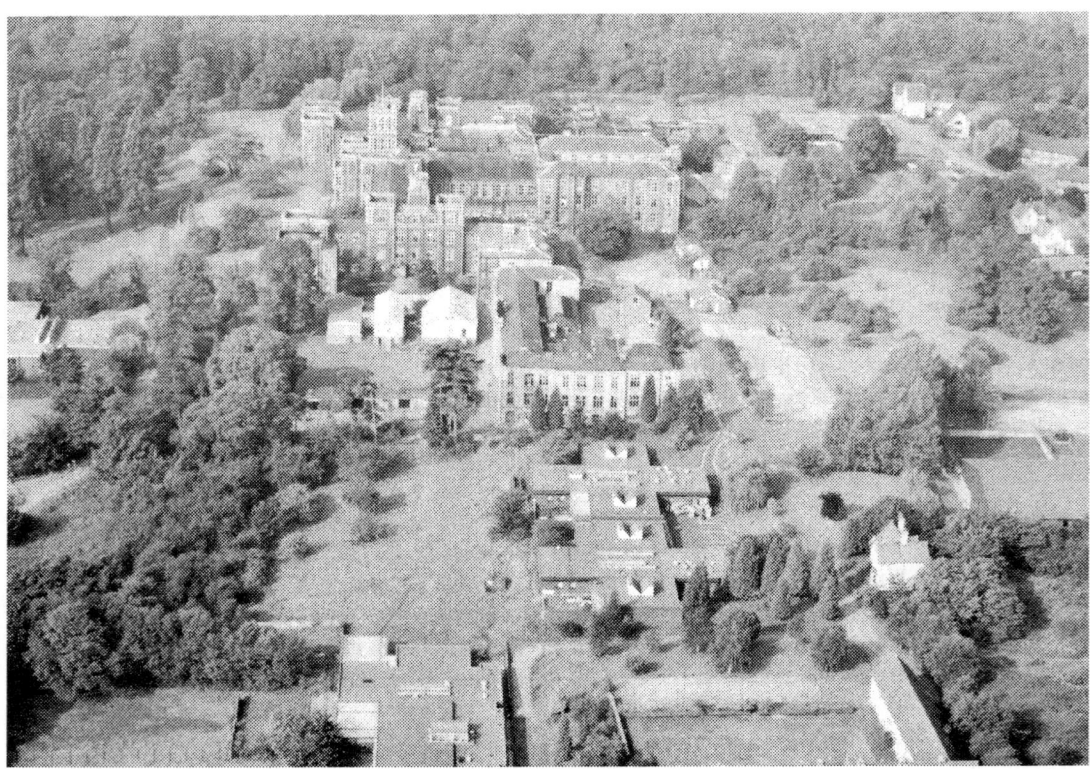

(Reprinted courtesy of J Street)

In 1927, a further act modified the definition of mental deficiency following an outbreak of Encephalitis Lethargica that left a number of children with disability. For the first time there

114

was recognition that facilities should reflect the needs of the individual. Emphasis was placed on the role of the local authority to supervise training and occupation. The responsibility that Andrew Reed felt for the care of the disabled was finally accepted by the state.

In 1929 the Wood Report recommended an increased use of community care, using such approaches as licence, halfway houses, guardianship etc. It also felt that the mental health services would benefit from greater co-ordination. By the time that Earlswood became part of the National Health Service in 1948 it was calculated that Learning Disability affected eight in every 1000 families.

There were controls to ensure that the residents of Earlswood were not held inappropriately. In the 1950's the Court of Quarter Sessions appointed 'Visitors of Institutions' in the county of Surrey. They visited every three months to see all those attaining the age of 21 years, plus any due for re-certification, to determine whether they should continue to be detained under order. In 1952 the Ministry of Health authorised short periods of care of up to eight weeks without certification. Although introduced in response to waiting lists and inadequate bed-space, this was a major departure in the treatment of the learning disabled. Previously, admission had generally led to a lifetime of care. 'Respite' care permitted individuals to live at home for longer by providing support to the families during periods of need.

The Royal Commission on the laws relating to Mental Illness and Mental Deficiency 1954-7 recommended the development of care in the community, hostels etc. The Hospital was to remain but patients were to be de-certified. They would remain on an informal basis. The Board of Control was to be abolished and mental health services were to be integrated into physical health services.

The Mental Health Act 1959 became law from the 1st of November 1960. The act made attendance at Junior Training Centres enforceable where it had previously been voluntary. The Board of Control was disbanded. On the occasion of their last inspection, the 'Visitors' recorded the following comment:

> **"Royal Earlswood Hospital has a long and unique history in the care and treatment of mental sub-normality at many different levels, and I am encouraged to feel, on the occasion of their <u>last visit</u> by a Commissioner of the Board of Control, that many years of devoted and enterprising service lie before it, in the same fine tradition."**
>
> **A.K. Ross, Comm. Board of Control**

In 1962 the Scott Report recommended improvements in the training of staff working in local health authority and hospital junior training centres. In 1971 the responsibility for these centres transferred from health to the education authorities. The Education (Handicapped Children) Act made education authorities responsible for providing schooling to all children including those with learning disability. This applied equally to schools within learning disability hospitals. In time these schools were to be relocated back into the community and integration was encouraged where appropriate to the needs of the child.

Employment.

It is often difficult to differentiate between those of low intelligence and those with a true learning disability. Some of the Earlswood residents showed a 'lopsided' development, being capable of some complex skills yet unable to care for themselves. The training given and the employment opportunities offered sought to build on the individual's strengths and develop their self-confidence. Any spontaneous interest was encouraged and extended if possible. It was hoped that, in this way, people could be prepared for a successful return to the wider world, with a realistic possibility of being able to earn an income and to take some responsibility for their own lives. Some of the residents had unexpected talents. For example, there was a shoemaker who was renown for his fantastic memory for history.

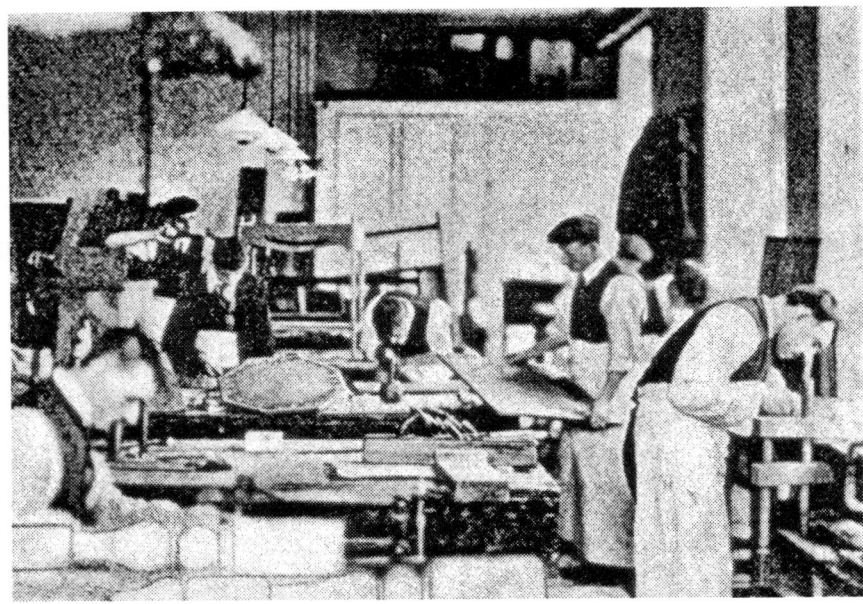

Woodcarvers

In 1862 there were already about 235 residents in useful employment within the Asylum. The carpenters were employed with woodcarving and cabinetwork.

> *There is a* "**carpenter shop....where one inmate proudly shews us a row of invalid chairs he has manufactured himself.**"

The mat weavers were making corridor matting, church matting and fancy mats. The tailors made clothes for all of the elected male residents as well as the attendants' uniforms.

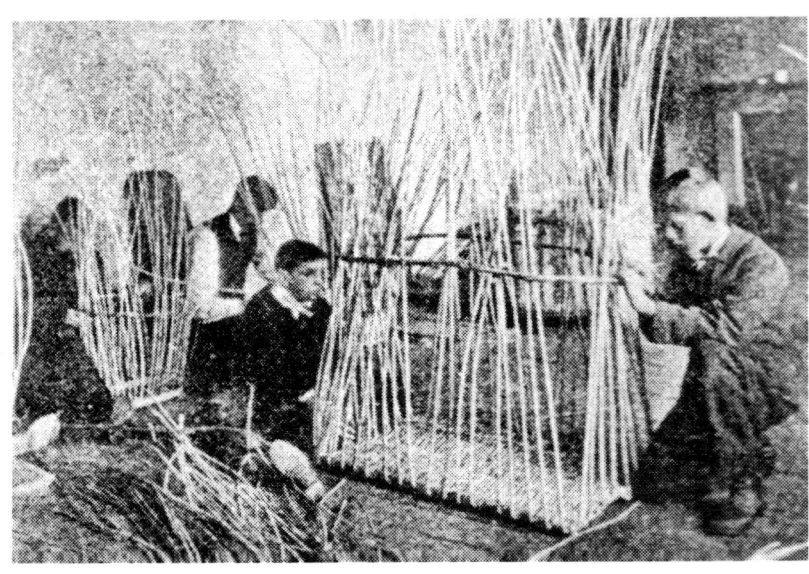

Basket making workshop

13 carpenters	12 shoemakers
82 mat weavers	7 basket weavers
10 tailors	1 bricklayer
20 farmworkers	6 laundry staff
24 girls and 14 boys at household work	
46 girls at needlework, lace making, bead mats etc.	

Employment of residents within Earlswood, 1862.

In only two years the range and number of posts available had increased as the talents of the residents and the needs of the Asylum changed. *'The Birmingham Post'*(i) in 1864 recorded the employment of 272 inmates.

18 carpenters	17 shoemakers
71 mat weavers	2 basket weavers
30 tailors	1 bricklayer
21 farmworkers	7 laundry staff
12 kitchen staff	1 postman
11 repairing clothes	4 assistant nurses
1 plumber	1 carrier
17 girls and 17 boys at household work	
41 girls at needlework, beadmats etc.	

Employment of residents within Earlswood, 1864.

In 1867 there was also a record of a baker and eleven shoe cleaners. The goal to provide useful employment for all continued. In a single year the total number of male residents increased by only one yet the number in employment expanded by 53. In 1875 there were 260 males and 105 women employed out of a total of 594 patients. This included 57 girls in industrial training, using all kinds of domestic skills such as cooking, cleaning, laundry etc. Fifteen thousand items were washed in the laundry weekly. Also mentioned were one turner, four printers, three painters, one blacksmith, two bakers, 16 gardeners, four men working in the wood yard, two store-men, two wardrobe staff, 27 bed-makers, five fancy goods makers, five

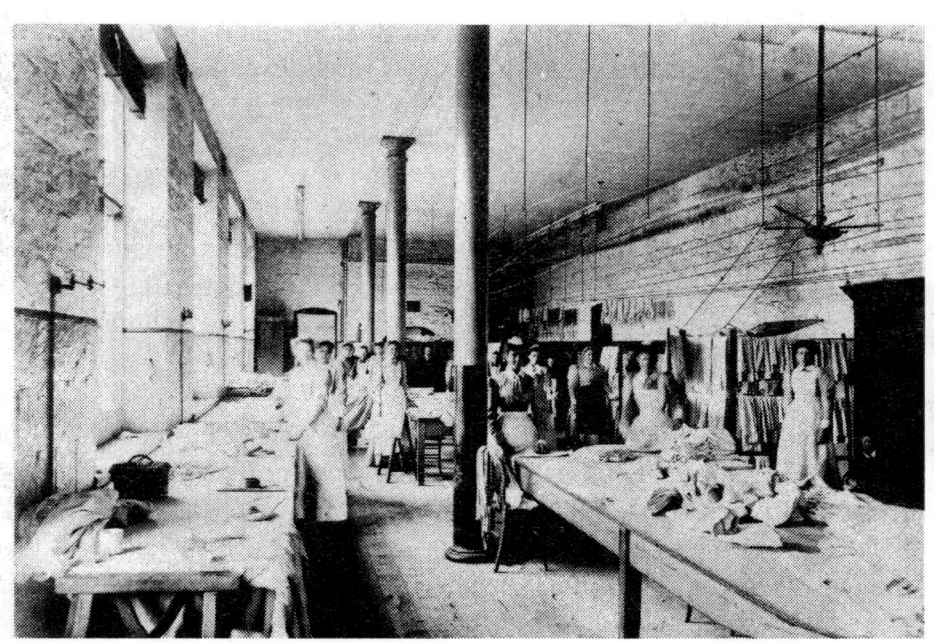

Laundry

(i)   Seventeen children had already been admitted from Birmingham and five were awaiting admission.

schoolroom monitors and one teacher, as well as all the other categories of staff previously mentioned. A new printing machine was purchased.

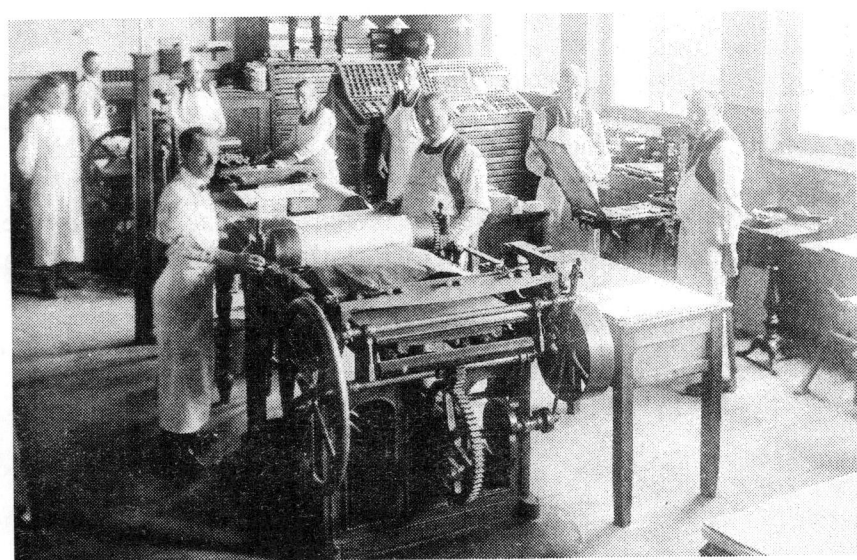

Print shop

Employment was recognised as bestowing self-value on the individual. In 1877 the tailors' shop made 881 garments at a profit of £77 3s 3d (£77-16p). In the shoemakers' shop 677 pairs of boots and shoes were made and a further 9118 pairs were repaired.

> **"Boot making room…. boot cleaners in red flannel jackets and black aprons….menders, sewers and welters are all doing useful work, under the superintendence of the master tradesman; and many a pluck at the coat-tails and constant offers to shake hands, and efforts to provoke our smiles, testifies to the supreme contentment of them all."**

In 1898 the print shop was the only workshop to accept outside orders. There were 232 private commissions, netting a profit of £150.

> **"….idiot carrier who drives his donkey cart down to the railway station daily, and brings all the parcels safely back, to the idiot postman who conveys all letter to and from the post without a single error."**

The report of the Commissioners of Lunacy recorded that 44% of men and 30% of women were usefully employed in 1904. In 1907 the shoemaking and tailoring workshops completed £900 worth of work, making 500 pairs of boots per year and all the clothes for the Asylum. The residents provided all the print work required by the Institution, including the List of Subscribers and the Annual Report. In 1908 the workshops were extended to allow many skilled crafts.

The *'Charity Record'* of the 30th of April 1910 reported that 171 of the residents were usefully employed. The residents of the Asylum produced baskets, hearthrugs, boots, shoes, clothes, fretwork frames, inkstands, brackets, carved tea trays and printed work. There were brushes for hats, hair, clothes, boots, scrubbing and crumbs, together with brooms of all sizes. Other inmates were employed in the laundry processing 12,000 to 13,000 items per week.

By 1952 there were 23 men employed on the farm, 16 in the market garden, 15 in the kitchen and 46 in the various workshops producing mats, boots, brushes, clothes, print work and upholstering furniture. Ten women were employed in the laundry helping with ironing and folding. Male patients distributed the clean laundry.

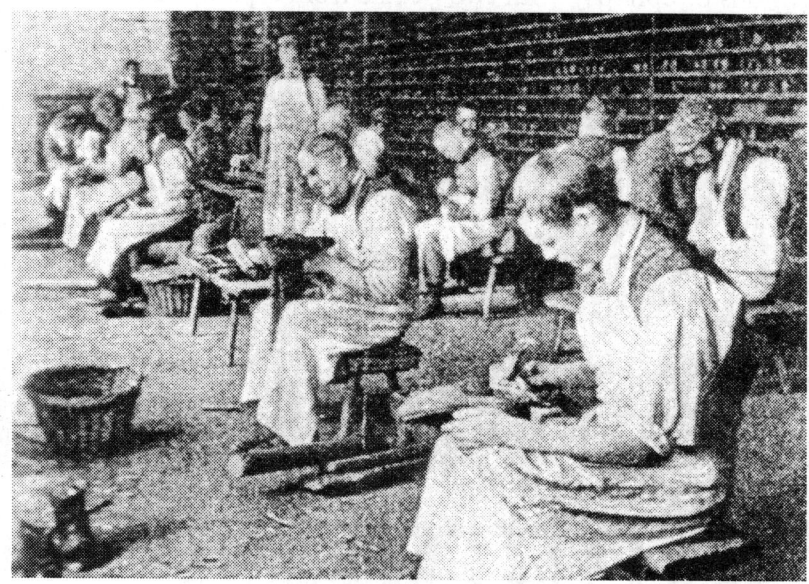

Cobblers' shop

A resident of Earlswood from 1942 until 1979 remembered first meeting Mr. Hooker, the printing 'shop-master'. He had asked for employment in this area. He learned how to operate the 'foot controlled treadle machines' and commented that they went so fast that he was afraid that the floor would give way. The working day was from 9a.m. until 11.45a.m. and 2p.m. until 4.30p.m. or 5p.m. when there was a task requiring urgent completion. The print shop produced all types of articles from X-ray request forms for the Redhill General Hospital to headed notepaper and compliment slips for each of the hospitals in the Royal Earlswood group. When the print shop-master retired the workshop was closed and the hospital printing went to an outside contractor. The same resident worked evenings on the hospital switchboard if the regular staff were ill.

In October 1972 the Thomas Parker Centre was opened by Sir Desmond Bonham-Carter, Chairman of the South West Metropolitan Regional Hospital Board. The Technical and Social Training Centre housed the Industrial Therapy Unit that had been built up over ten years. Employment was provided there for some residents, in direct competition with outside contractors. Work included packing of cosmetics and of spray paint, checking terminals for micro batteries, sorting and grading gemstones for jewellery and carpentry – making chessboard, plant troughs and nesting boxes.

Numbers

The number of people requiring the kind of care and education offered by the Charity quickly outstripped the space at Park House and a second Asylum had to be established at Essex Hall. In 1849 Park House accommodated 66 residents, by April 1852 there were 141 in the two locations.

By 1857, with the new building at Earlswood finally completed and the lease at Park House ended, the average occupation between Redhill and Colchester reached 274. In 1861-2 there were 231 males and 100 females cared for at Earlswood. There were sixty new admissions that year with 31 being discharged, 29 of whom were recorded as having made some improvement.

Seven men and 5 women went on to find employment; the former as tailors, mat makers and a carpenter, while the later became domestic servants. Twenty-one inmates died in the same year, mainly from pulmonary conditions or epilepsy with two deaths from typhoid fever.

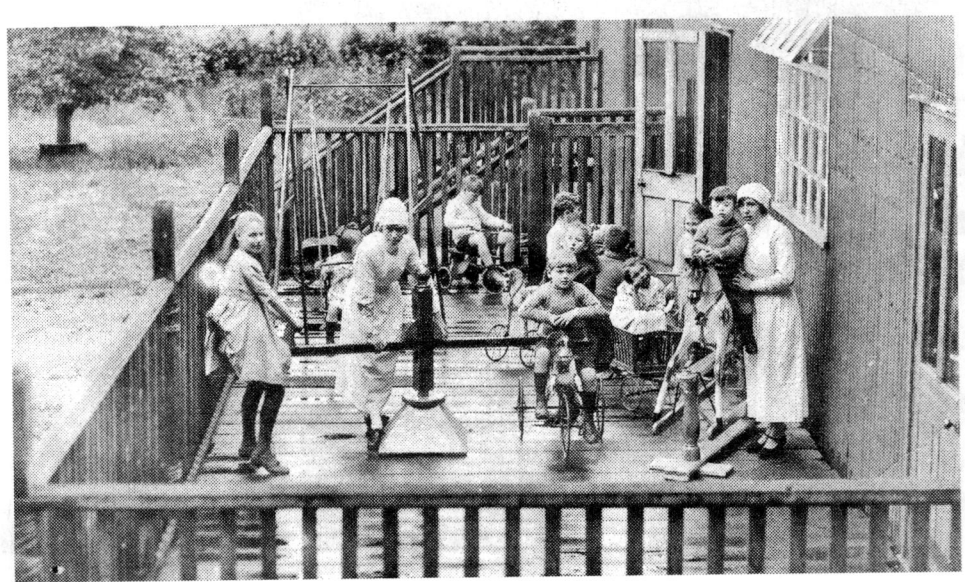

A children playground

In 1863 there were 18311 idiots identified in England with 350 housed at Earlswood. This increased to 365 in 1864 with 130 full paid places and the rest admitted by election. Earlswood now accepted all ages and in 1865 there were 66 men, 34 women, 133 boys, 67 girls and 100 infants cared for within its walls. Numbers were increasing steadily during this period, 446 in 1866, 476 by 1868, 1870 saw the population top 500. However, there were times when shortage of money prevented Earlswood accepting as many election cases as it could have accommodated.

The 1871 census in England and Wales listed 29,452 idiots. Earlswood in 1874 accommodated 385 males and 191 females, of whom 100 had been admitted for life. In 1875 a further 129 were admitted whilst 49 were discharged and 30 died, generally from epilepsy or chest complaints.

Altogether, 295 male and 106 female inmates were usefully employed within the Institution. Over the next few years numbers stabilised and even fell slightly due to financial constraints. In 1877 there were 609 inmates. In 1878 only 52 were admitted whilst 44 were discharged and 34 died, 26 of these below the age of 20 and the oldest were two women both aged 40. A man of 24 died in an unfortunate accident when he was hit by a railway engine.

By 1880 the number within Earlswood had fallen to 562 but over 2000 had passed through its doors since the Charity was founded. The Board recorded that 17 had been cured, 730 improved, 145 had not benefited, whilst 502 had died. As funding improved numbers again increased, by 1891 reaching an average through the year of 635. The problems with the deterioration of the building, encountered in the early 20th century, forced the Asylum to reduce its numbers. Although much of the reconstruction work progressed without relocating the residents, there was an inevitable effect on the number that could safely be accommodated. The dust and damp resulting from the work also increased the number of deaths from pneumonia and chest complaints. In 1906 it was noted that 4000 had been treated at Earlswood since its beginning, the Asylum could hold 650 but the state of building limited the occupancy to 427.

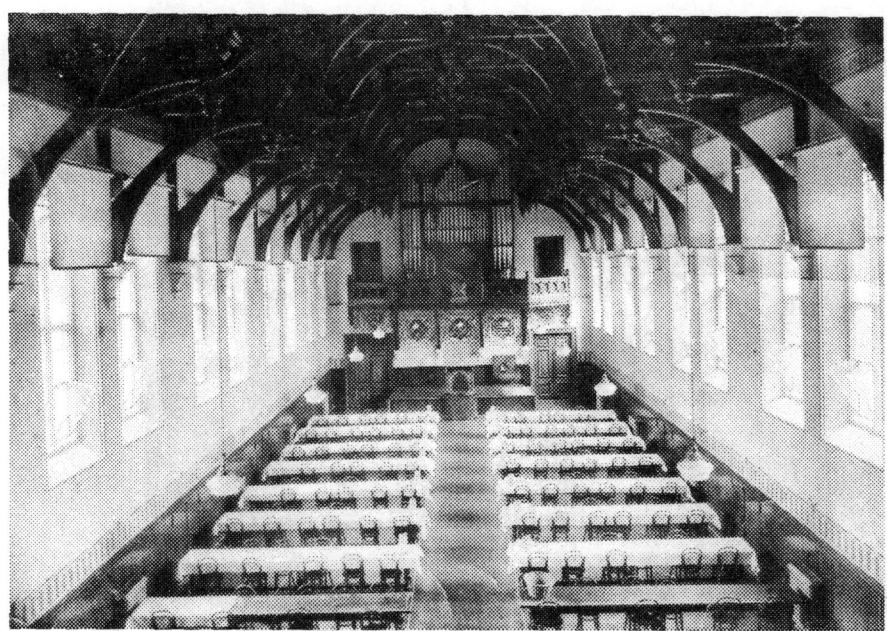

The main hall

In 1908 it was noted that mortality was running at no more than 4% of the population, an improvement on the figure of 4.6% recorded in 1883. Given the difficulty of carrying out major building work this provides evidence of the high level of care achieved. Fifty-three inmates had been resident for more than 40 years and 17 for over 50 years. The population in 1909 included 267 who had been admitted without payment, 108 had paid up to 65 guineas, 25 paid between 65 and 250 guineas, seven paid above this figure and life payment had been received for 34.

By 1911 residency had increased a little to 466. Forty-five people were elected in the usual way together with 12 additional candidates who had been unsuccessful at four consecutive elections; this concession was made in honour of the coronation of George V. The records showed that 87 people had been resident in Earlswood for more than 30 years, 52 for over 40 years, 19 over 50 years and one resident for in excess of 60 years. The latter was almost certainly James Henry Pullen who initial admission had been to Essex Hall. The Board was pleased to report that one resident of 18 years was so improved that he was now a farm foreman superintendent in South Africa.

The numbers did not increase during the war years. This was probably due to the ongoing restoration work, the loss of attendants to the Front and the depletion of charitable funds in a country committed to a 'total war'. Indeed, it was not until the late 1920s that occupancy again reached 500. Thereafter growth was slow and numbers in Earlswood did not top the 600 mark until 1952, four years after it became part of the National Health Service. At that time the Earlswood Group of three hospitals, Forest, Farmfield and Earlswood could accommodate 1120 in total with the latter having a total of 606 inmates, 396 males and 210 females.

Maximum occupancy was reached in the 1960s with around 675 being permanently accommodated, 60% of whom were male. With the addition of the Villas Earlswood could accommodate a maximum of 706 residents but some beds were now being used for respite purposes, temporary care of community clients to give their families a break or during periods of illness or crisis. In addition, Forest Hospital could treat 370, Farmfield 180 and there were 28 beds at the holiday home at Walton-on-the-Naze, giving a total of 1284 beds.

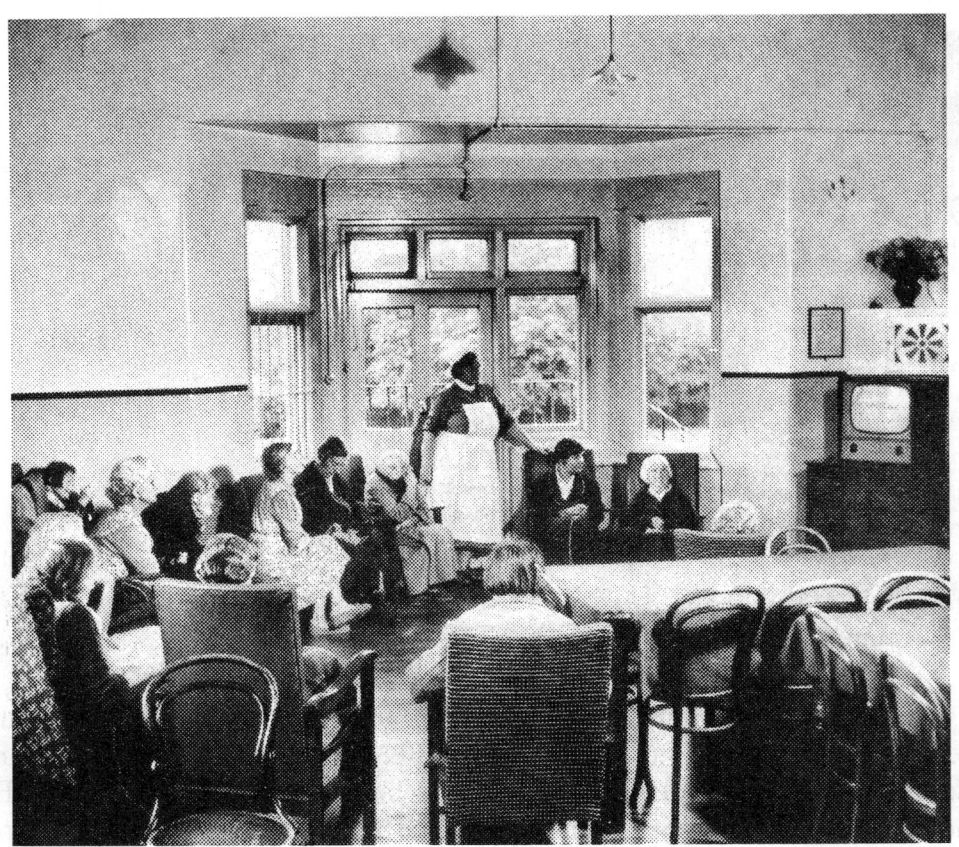

A ward

There were no significant changes to the numbers receiving care at Earlswood during the 1970s. However, by the 1980s attitudes to residential care began to change. Children with a Mental Handicap began to be educated in the community and were no longer admitted to Earlswood except for respite. The 1990s saw the major change with the idea of Care in the Community put into action in a major way. By 1994 there were only about 290 permanent residents in Earlswood and the respite provision for the children had moved into the community. In 1996 numbers had fallen to a little over 230 and in the month before the final closure of Earlswood the last 120 residents were finally placed in their new community homes.

Outings.

From the earliest days the residents of Earlswood enjoyed excursions to educational exhibitions as well as outings to the seaside. In September 1865 a party of 76 boys and 35 girls visited the exhibition at Crystal Palace, accompanied by the schoolmaster, the girls' governess and six teachers. The London, Brighton and South Coast Railway Company provided special carriages at a discount and the management of Crystal Palace offered reduced price tickets. The residents paid the remaining costs. The Medical Superintendent, Dr. Down took a further 150 pupils to Crystal Palace in the following year. In August 1867 an even larger group of 200 residents enjoyed the spectacular exhibition. A similar number attended in August 1868 accompanied by the new Medical Superintendent Dr. Grabham. He recorded:

'...a thoroughly happy day was spent; the conduct of all the pupils was exemplary. The expenses were defrayed by small voluntary contributions from the friends of the inmates. The amount sent, in answer to an appeal, exceeded by several pounds what was required: and the balance was placed in our Savings bank, to the credit of a number of pupils.'

In 1878 a party of 29 men visited Crystal Palace.

Suitable inmates enjoyed holidays at home with their families and this assisted their general improvement. However, this was not possible for many and an annual summer excursion provided an opportunity for the less fortunate to enjoy a change of environment. On the 9th of August 1870 the annual excursion was to Portslade. Two hundred and eighty people, including 27 staff, enjoyed the outing. The residents rose at five in the morning and breakfasted at 5.45am. A special train left Redhill at 7.15am. On arrival the entire party walked to the beach. They had meat sandwiches and lemonade and two boats were provided to row small parties around the harbour. Cricket was played on the green and in the afternoon 100 boys bathed. An entry in the schoolmaster's journal records that they 'took three dozen towels and six combs'. They also included 24 spades for building sand castles. Mr. Gahegan took his cornet to 'sound the calls'.

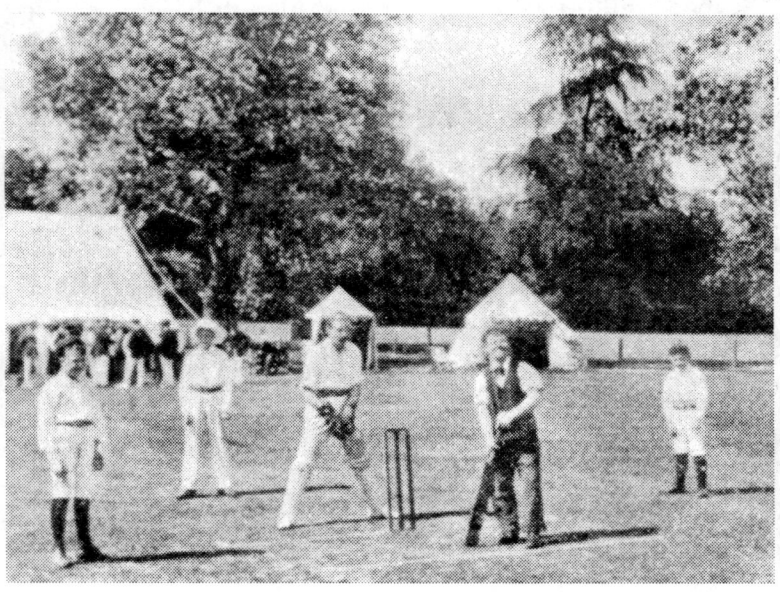

A cricket match

After this tea was served before the party walked back to the station at 6.30pm to catch the train at 7.31pm. The happy revellers arrived home at 9.20pm and enjoyed supper in the hall before falling exhausted into their beds. In 1871 the outing on the 8th of August was to Seaford. Special carriages were provided on the train to accommodate the 285 residents and 47 staff. The Friends of the Asylum provided funds for the trip. On the return trip the train was halted specially at Earlswood to allow the trippers to disembark. On the 24th of July 1874 staff together with 418 out of a total of 569 residents enjoyed a day trip to Littlehampton. Always supportive of the Asylum, the London, Brighton and South Coast Railway laid on a special train paid for by friends and relatives.

According to the schoolmaster's journal another outing was made to the Wombwell Menagerie at Redhill. The party was made up of 59 females and 130 males, with six female and 10 male attendants, together with 13 officers. They paid three pence halfpenny (1.5p) per head.

After the war 'daily parole' was introduced for some of the male residents. They would go out, in groups of three, the most able or responsible being nominated as the leader. Generally they would enjoy an afternoon outing to Redhill for shopping, tea or perhaps a visit to the cinema.

Outings became a regular part of the daily life. The Hospital obtained a coach and there were two trips organised every week. In October 1972 the Variety Club of Great Britain presented a Sunshine Coach to the Hospital. A second one followed in August 1978. Costing £5,000, it was sponsored by Keith Prowse and Co. Ltd. The entertainments listed in the Annual Report for 1973 include coach trips, concerts, dances, outing, cinema visits, river trips, clubs and visits to shops. The Hospital provided the vast majority of entertainment and excursions for the residents with only five to ten percent of them receiving regular visits from family or friends.

In 1979 there were regular outings on Sundays for the children. The residents of Victoria and Philip homes, together with three children from Andrew Reed, were out from 9.15am and 11.30am and the remaining children from Andrew Reed plus those from Elizabeth and Mark homes enjoyed their excursion between 2pm and 4pm.

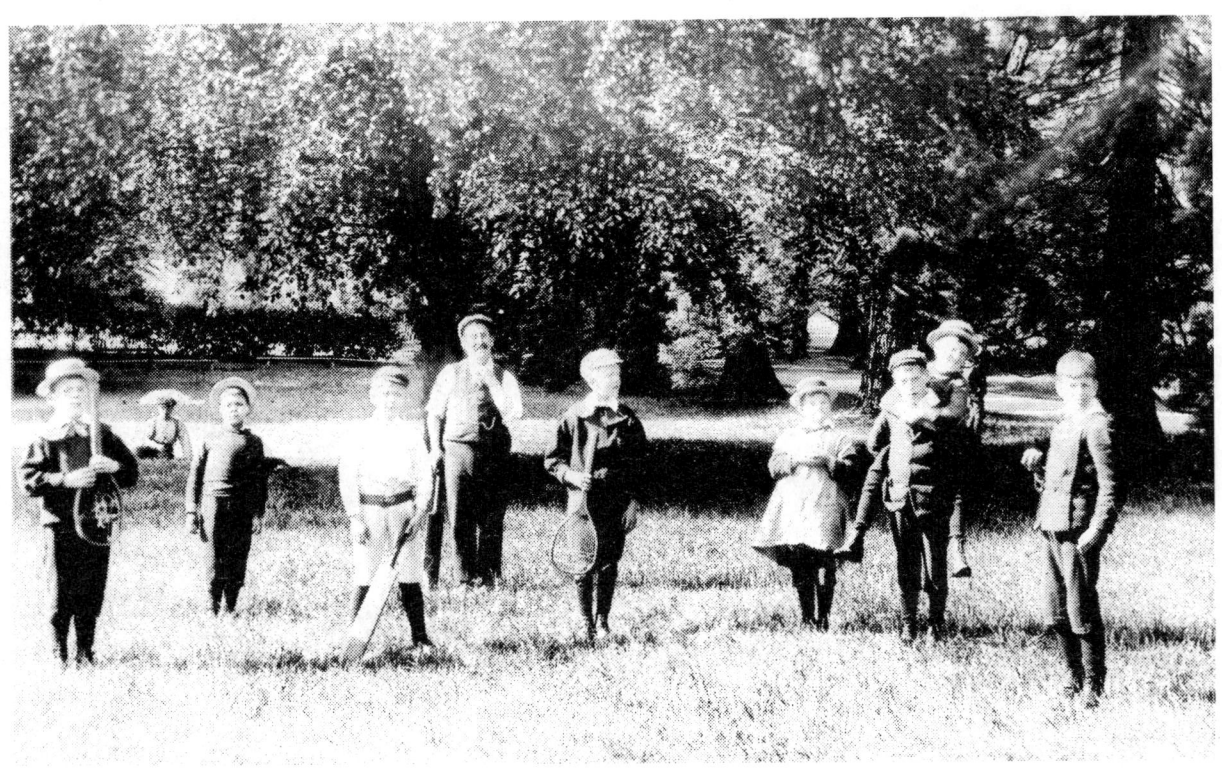

Boys at play

Farming

From the very beginning the value of outdoor activity and good food was recognised. In 1853 seven acres of kitchen garden was laid out and 35 cows were kept to provide milk for the residents of the Asylum. Aviaries were constructed, as well as several miles of walks. By 1862 there were two attendants and over 20 boys working on the farm, which had 24 cows, a new cow house and dairy. A further acre of land was purchased with accommodation for farm servants.

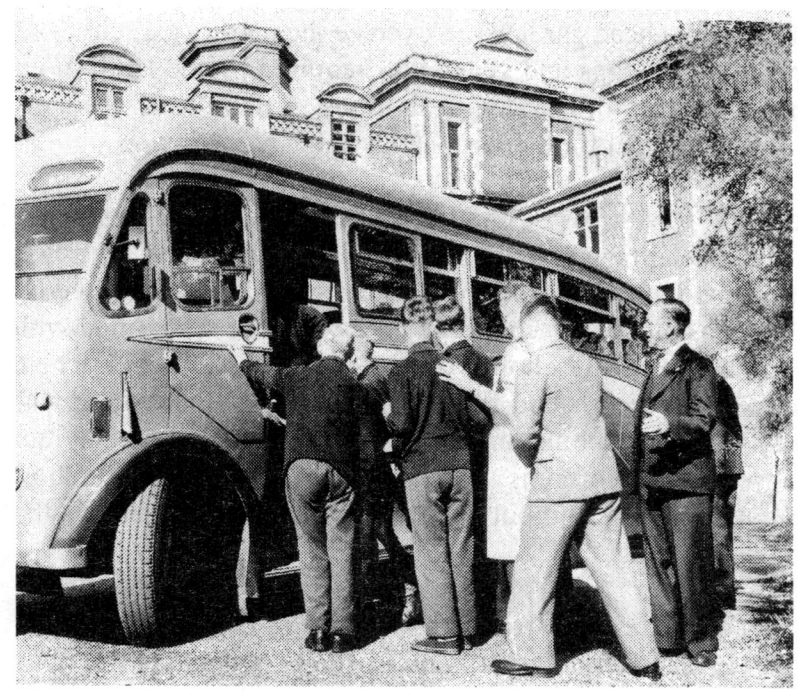

An outing

The Board agreed that there was a need to develop the most up to date farm buildings. In January 1873 the Board approved the site chosen for the new farm buildings and authorised plans to be drawn up. The plans were submitted in March 1873 and accepted. The House Committee was instructed to proceed with the project. Members of the Board and six of their friends made a special contribution of £1,483-10s-0d (£1,483.50) for the new farm buildings. By February 1874 the new buildings were almost complete and two members of the House Committee, Messr. Westall and Kelsey, were chosen to superintend the future arrangements of the farm and the estate generally and to report back to the Board on occasion. The Steward, Mr. Brown, was instructed to communicate with them before making any purchases for the farm.

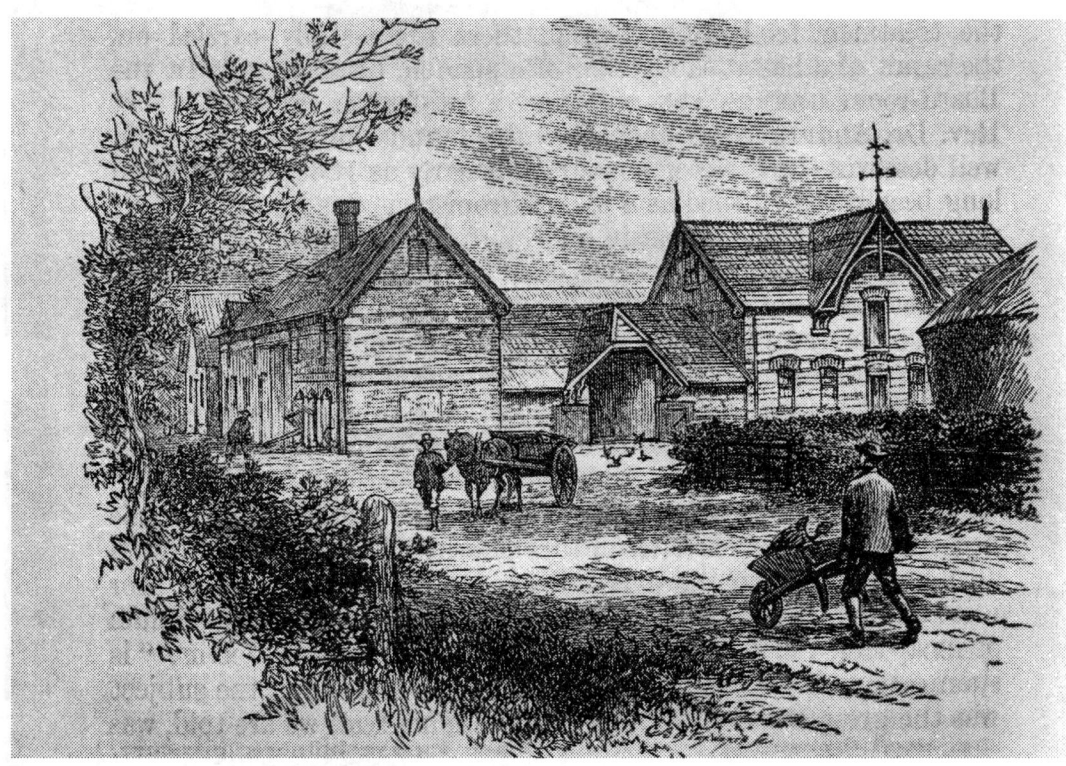

The farm

There was a bailiff to manage the farm and a head gardener to oversee the market gardens. The farm supplied most of the milk, meat, butter, eggs and vegetables required by the Institution, thus the residents and staff were ensured plenty of healthy, fresh foods. A number of residents worked on the farm and there was an annual treat for the farm hands and haymakers.

The farm buildings were extended in 1876 with barns, granaries, stables, dairies and pigsties. There was also a cart shed, a store and an engine house. The roof was in Bridgewater tiles with alternate rows of red and brown. The cow house had iron troughs and stall fittings supplied by James Burton of Oxford Street. Water was piped to each trough. The windows were fitted with regulating louver boarding. There was a new bailiff's house comprising a living room, kitchen, scullery, bacon room and dairy scullery on the ground floor, with a dairy at the rear. It was designed by J Brown, the steward, and J.G Gibbins, architect, and erected by the Asylum workmen. On the first floor there were four bedrooms. By this stage the farm had 40 short horned cattle and 120 pigs. The entire sewage output of the Asylum was spread on the grassland and was beneficial in periods of drought.

The farm was run for many years as a separate entity from the Asylum. A charge of £300 per annum was made on the farm and garden account in lieu of rent. In 1874 the value of the stock was assessed at £1,859. This was transferred to the farm committee and entered into the Asylum accounts as a loan. Interest of five percent was charged until 1899, at which point it

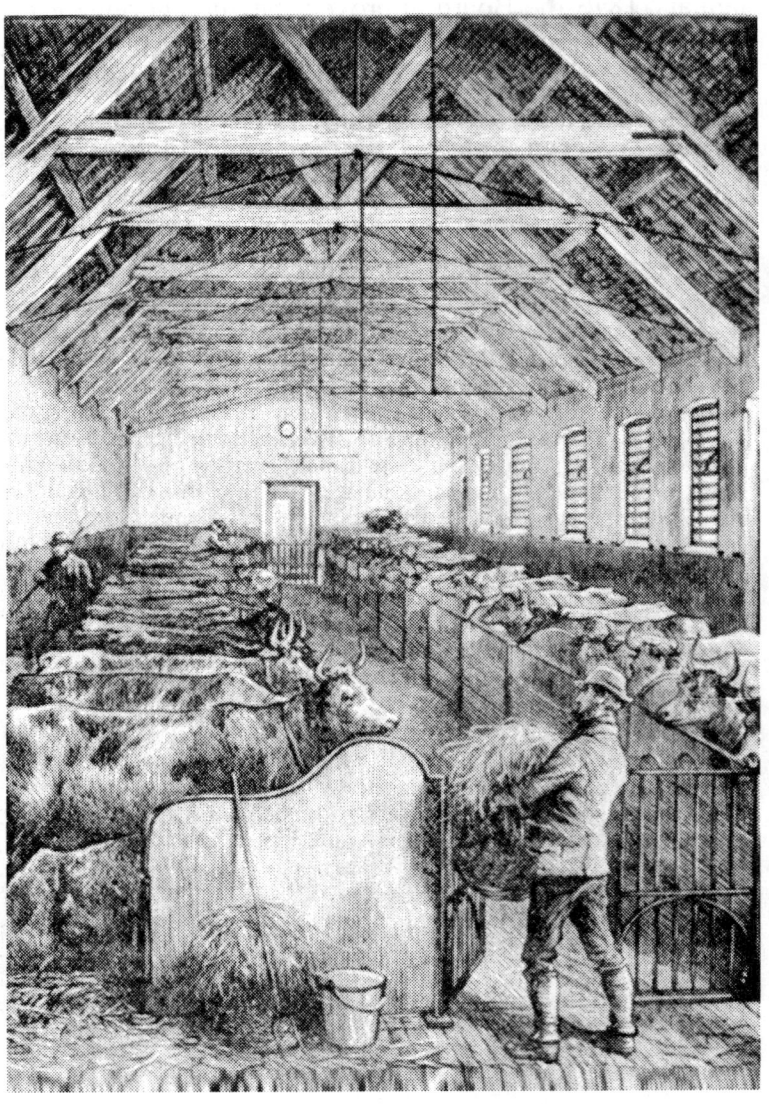

The cattle byre

was discontinued. The Hospital purchased the food it required from the farm and for the first few years any profits that were made were passed to housekeeping. This offset the cost of provisions thus bringing down charges to approximately cost price.

In 1879 the Horley Mead, a further 25 acres, were purchased to permit increased production. The purchase price of £4,000 was borrowed from the General Assurance Company, to be repaid over ten years. In 1887 additional land known as Ireland's Brickyard and field was purchased for £2,100 out of existing funds. The farm was required to pay Holmes' tithes every year at a cost of £20. In 1894 a sum was paid to redeem the tithes, cancelling the need for all future payments. In 1889 £800 from the farm account was used to build farm cottages in Princes Road and in 1899 a further £600 was used for further cottages in Hooley Road. Additional cottages were built on Ireland's field though the date is unclear as no record appears in the farm account. Although the farm had expanded greatly there had been no increase in the rent charged, indeed, in 1881 and 1889 the bad harvests had resulted in a half years rent being excused.

As a result of the above the housekeeping account between 1886 and 1902 received only £1,400, compared to £6,543 between 1874 and 1885. Without profits to offset the charges made by the farm for provisions there were complaints about the cost to housekeeping. However, the farm argued that it could sell the food at a higher price elsewhere. This was one of the factors that induced the Board to instigate an investigation into the way the farm finances were managed. The report was produced in 1902.

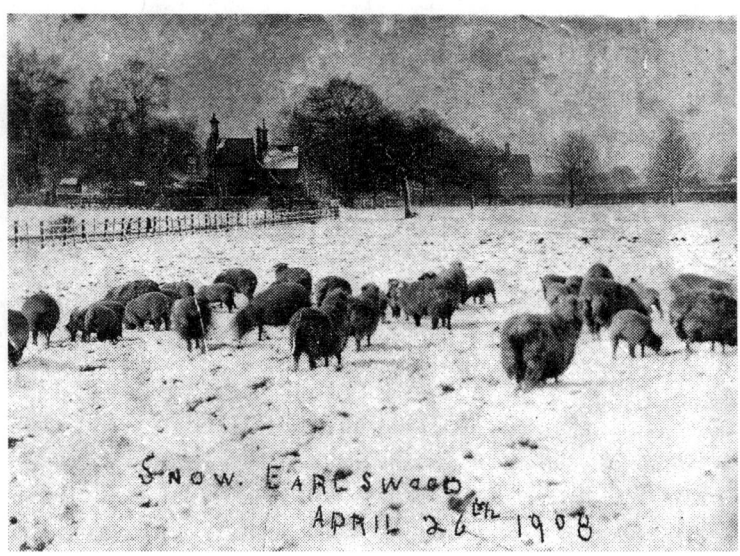

The farm committee was found to have acted unilaterally and to have kept no proper accounts. They had made decisions and drawn cheques without reference to the Board. Gratuities of £20 and £10 had been paid at Christmas each year to the Steward and the Farm Bailiff respectively. No stock books had been kept and there were no detailed accounts of goods sold and income earned. The auditors were unhappy with matters and recommended that "proper accounts should be kept by the London Office". It argued that the farm existed to produce good, cheap food, not to make a profit. The price of food production exceeded that at the other Asylums in the country.

The Hospital required 66 gallons of milk a day but production varied from 70 to 82 gallons per day depending on the time of year. The garden was running at a loss and the report recommended pensioning off the manager.

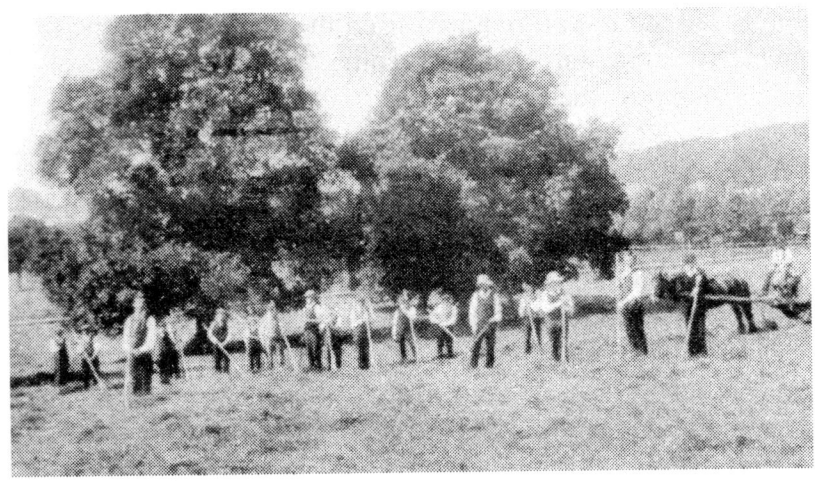

Haymaking

Mr. Wells was farm bailiff and his son then became bailiff in his own right from about 1900 to 1950. There was a cowman, a carter, a pig man and a shepherd. The head cowman received £1 –1s –0p (£1.05p) per week out of which he paid four shillings (20pence) a week in rent. He had a garden and as much in the way of vegetables as he needed and would receive a shilling (5 pence) for every calf born alive. The pig man would receive a similar sum for each farrow of pigs. The head carter received a pound and the second carter 19 shillings (95 pence) per day. The asylum was charged 25 shillings (£1.25 pence) per day for man and cart.

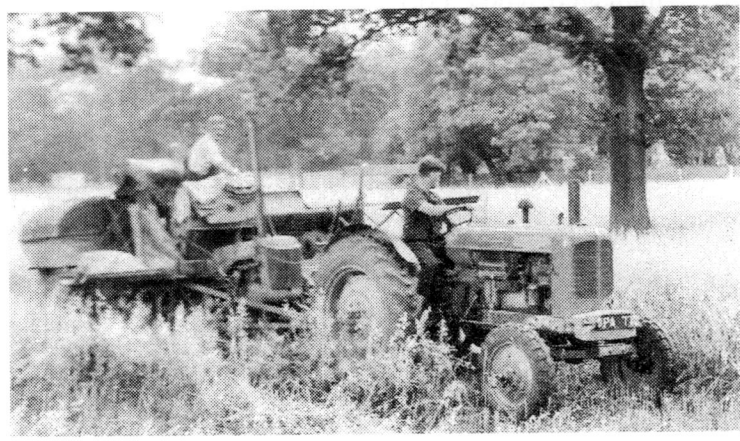

On the farm

Mr. Terry lived in a separate cottage at the bottom of the estate and received a pound in pay. Mr. Brown was employed as fencer and general odd job man. Mr. Peters was the top man and lived in the lodge. He received £1-7s (£1.35 pence) per day and was in charge of several men and six to eight garden boys.

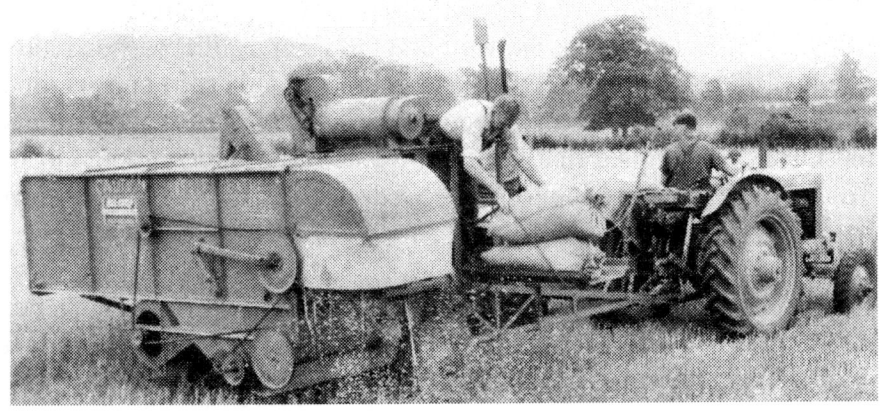

Farm production

On the farm there were no holidays. The cowman, with the help of eight to ten boys, looked after a dairy herd of 50 to 65 cows necessary to keep the yield of milk up to a suitable level. The animals were fed and milked by hand. The milk was tipped into big cans and taken to the kitchen where some was made into butter for the officers. It was made into pats with a cow or pheasant embossed on them. The dairy staff were "in major trouble with matron" if the task was not carried out satisfactorily.

The farm produced 200 tons of potatoes per years. There were 150-200 pigs. Every two weeks two pigs, three sheep and one bullock would be killed to supply meat to the Asylum. One member of the farm staff remembered that, every morning he would go across the lawn and under the three arches to a pub called the 'Nag's Head'. There he would have a half pint of beer costing one penny (0.5p)

By 1906 Earlswood had 108 acres of land with over 100 acres given over to the farm and market gardens, providing much of the food for the 800 residents and staff. In 1908 the farm won many prizes at the Redhill and Reigate agricultural show. In 1911 Mr. Wells achieved first class awards for pigs, hay, potatoes etc. at the same show. The hospital museum collection includes a cup inscribed 'Redhill Fat Stock Show 1929' though it is unknown precisely for what the prize was awarded.

In 1925 the Rt. Hon. Earl de la Warr was elected to the Board bringing with him expertise on farming. The farm, at this time, had 130 acres. There were 40 shorthorn cattle and rear bullocks plus sheep. There was a kitchen garden and the farm produced the majority of the fodder needed for the animals. It also supplied all the milk and eggs required by the residents. In the late 1920s an additional 33 cows were purchased at a cost of approximately £36 each. Thirty store pigs, aged 12-20 weeks, were acquired at 50-55 shillings (£2.50-£2.75) each.

By 1948/9 the total area of land being farmed for the Royal Earlswood Hospital Group included 160 acres of arable and 130 acres of pasture. There were four acres of market garden. Nearly 188 acres were farmed at Burford and Lonesome Farms. The commercial herd of dairy cows was sold and replaced by a herd of attested Friesians. In 1950 the dairy and cowshed were modified.

In 1951 a new bullpen was built. The Hospital dairy herd was increased from 65 to 114 and the number of pigs from 69 to 117. In addition there were nine fat cows and 112 bacon pigs produced for the Ministry of Food. The Royal Earlswood Hospital Group was farming approximately 700 acres in four estates at Earlswood, Farmfield, Lonesome Lane and Burford

In 1952 a Dutch barn was erected at the farm on Lonesome Lane. Twenty-three men were employed on the farm and 16 in the market gardens. In 1959 the Lonesome and Burford estates were sold, reducing the Hospital farm by 180 acres. Farming continued at Royal Earlswood and Farmfield, a total of approximately 500 acres, worked by 23 men. Pigpens were built at Royal Earlswood allowing increased production. In November 1961 a fire destroyed the pig farrowing unit and the entire stock but this was quickly rebuilt. A covered cattle yard was developed at Farmfield. All milk had now to be sold to the Milk Marketing Board from which the Hospital purchased its needs. The Hospital had sufficient cattle to ensure that there were 45 in milk at any one time. Silos were purchased for the drying of grain. Iron boundary fencing can still be found marking the extent of the estate at Earlswood.

	Meat	Milk	Cream	Eggs	Fowl	Potatoes
	lbs	gal	pt	doz		lbs
1937	28,700	27,951		623.5	799.5lbs	101,452
1938	29,732	27162	12	1,687	239 head	91,336
1939	29,412	29,009	30.5	2,384	403 head	70,812
1940	26,310	23,659	27	1,756	465 head	63,961
1941	7,868	21,673		1,501	162 head	125,440
1942	0	19,963		264.25	42 head	134,400
1943	0	19,641		261.3	21 head	156,800
1944	0	20,491		104	181 head	153,888
1945	0	26,342		167	53lbs geese	175,840
1946	0	23,735		99.5	54lbs geese	184,576
1947	0	22,974		81		78,848
1948	0	18,053		46.5		103,331
1951		23,000			200pullets/180 cockrells/40 geese	
1952	49,000 (122 cattle/215 pigs)				200 head	
1953	300 pigs	25,112				
1954		25,417		2,374		
1956	684 pigs	51,100				
1957	721 pigs 18,955lb beef	38,300				
1958	597 pigs					
1962	60 dairy cows, 180 pigs	51,100				

	Swede + greens	Tomato	Beetroot	Apples	Fruit/Veg
	lbs	lbs	lbs	lbs	£ - s - d
1937	15,695				225-13- 7
1938	17,149				335-12- 6
1939	16,125				420- 2- 1
1940	8,504	2,764			659-13- 2
1941	17,668				762-18- 6
1942	36,864		5,035		606-19- 5
1943	44,028		5,578		601-12- 4
1944	62,202	3,843	2,700	4,409	406- 5- 1
1945	57,883	2,628	8,757	7,588	458-13-10
1946	62,841	1,552.5	11,480	6,816	362- 6- 6
1947	49,661	3,120	8,886	6,706	397- 2- 7
1948	63,655	2,603	6,944	4,339	297- 9-10
1951					self sufficient in vegetables
1954					2,600-0-0

Production on Royal Earlswood Farm from 1937-1962.
(Gaps indicate a lack of information not necessarily of production.)

By 1962 there were 400 acres under cultivation, with 180 pigs in production and 160 milk cows producing 140 gallons of milk per day. However, in 1964 the farm was finally closed as a result of a government decision that this type of employment no longer had a part to play in the life of the residents of long-stay hospitals.

Christmas and the Winter Entertainments

Christmas Day started early at Earlswood. Each nursery and parlour would have a prettily decorated tree. The residents were awoken by music at 5.45am, often carol singers touring the homes. After breakfast the medical superintendent would do his round, greeting all. Letters,

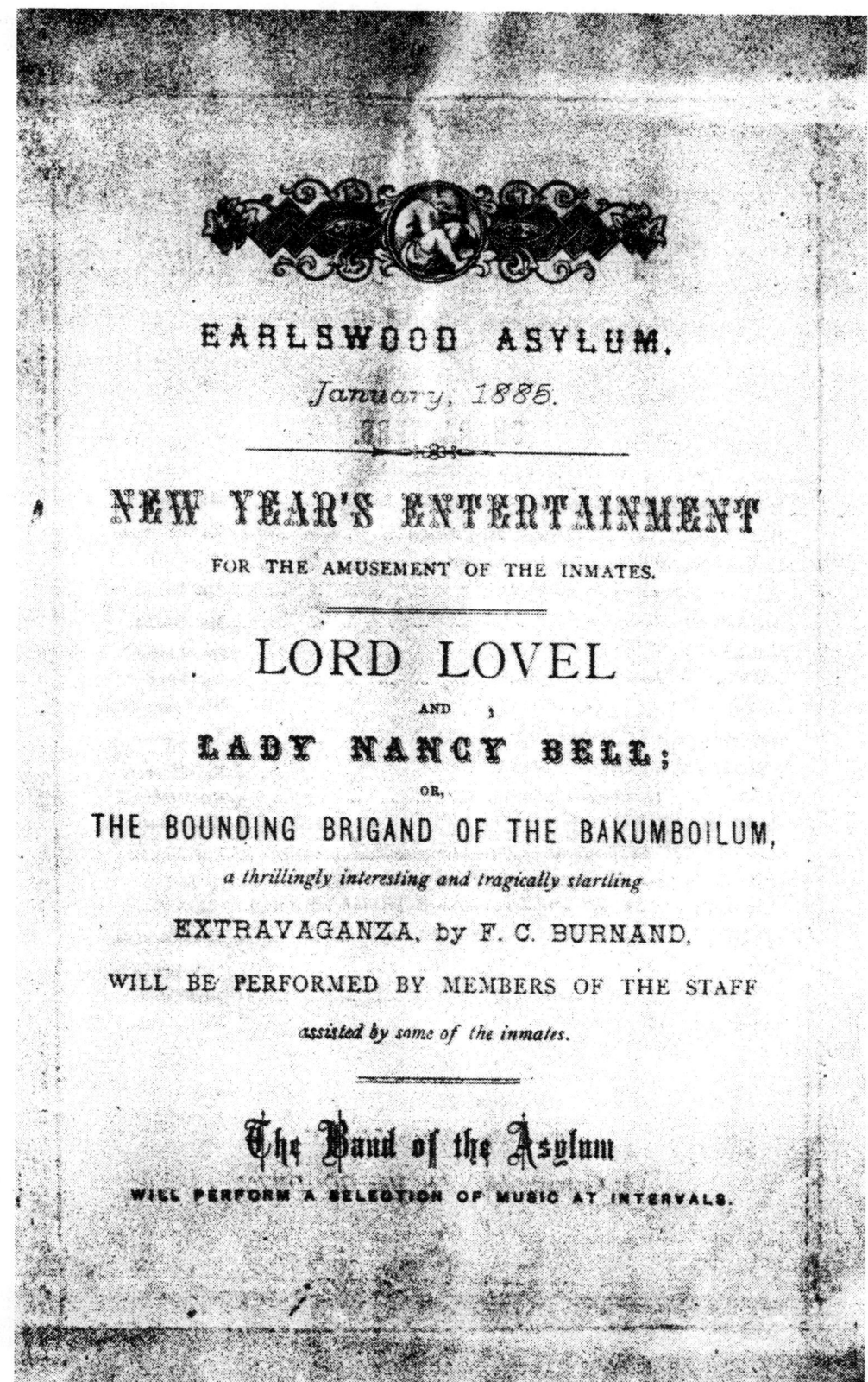

EARLSWOOD ASYLUM.

January, 1885.

NEW YEAR'S ENTERTAINMENT

FOR THE AMUSEMENT OF THE INMATES.

LORD LOVEL

AND

LADY NANCY BELL;

OR,

THE BOUNDING BRIGAND OF THE BAKUMBOILUM,

a thrillingly interesting and tragically startling

EXTRAVAGANZA, by F. C. BURNAND,

WILL BE PERFORMED BY MEMBERS OF THE STAFF

assisted by some of the inmates.

The Band of the Asylum

WILL PERFORM A SELECTION OF MUSIC AT INTERVALS.

hampers and packages from family and friends would then be distributed. In 1910 there were 300 letters on Christmas Day, which was celebrated on Monday the 26th of December. As midday approached a huge Yule Log would be taken around by a group of residents in costume. They carried a collecting box and the proceeds were divided between them. At 12.30pm Christmas dinner would be served, roast beef produced from the Asylum's own farm. The Yule Log would be dragged into the centre of the dining room by a troop of patients led by

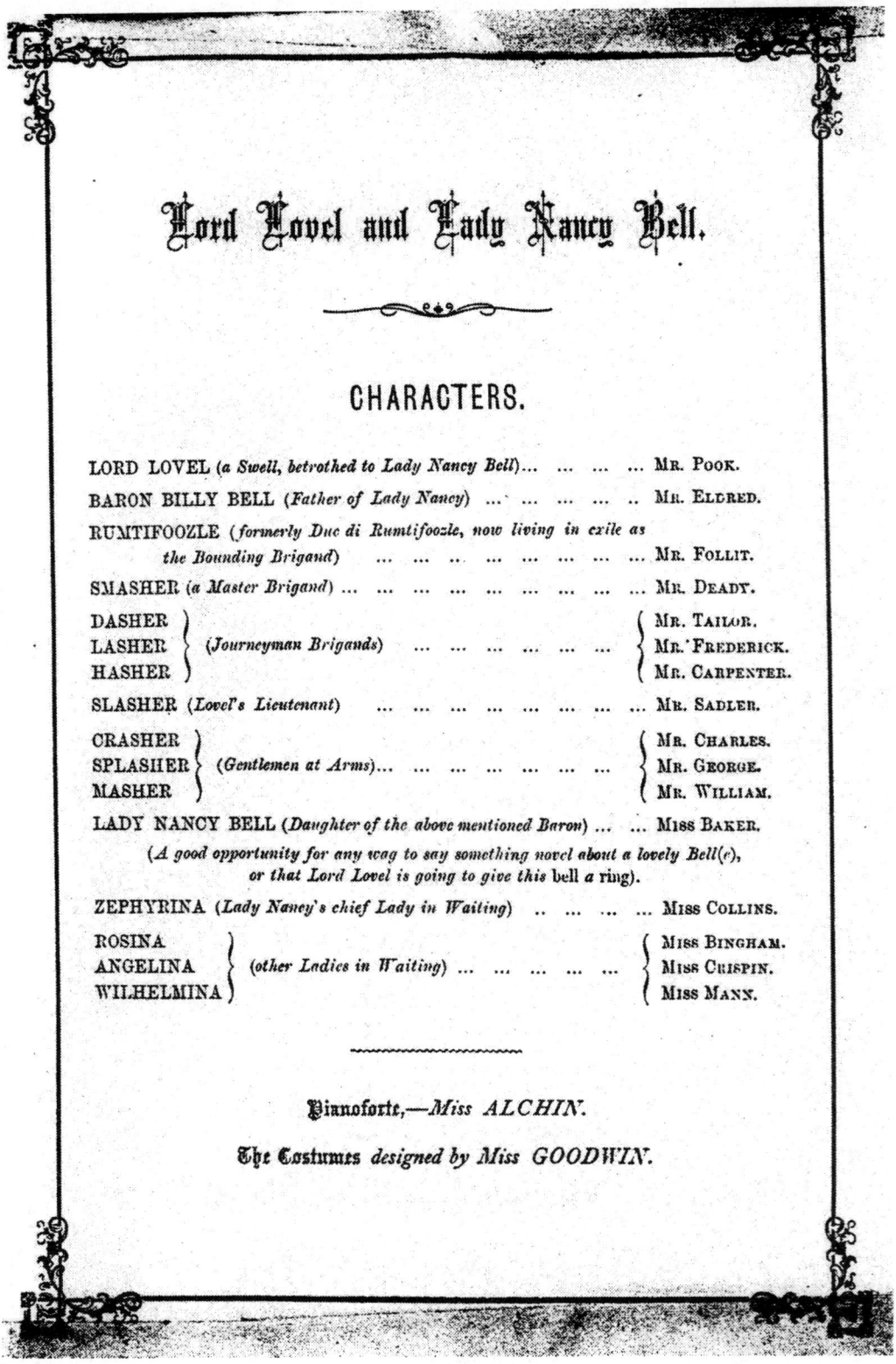

New Year's Entertainment program

the Asylum's oldest resident dressed in a cook's outfit and balancing a giant plum pudding on his head. Wagons bearing plates of Christmas fare followed. At 4pm a service of carols and readings would take place. The happy but exhausted residents were no doubt ready for bed following tea at 5.30pm. The attendants and servants were then free to enjoy their own dinner and celebrations. The entertainment at Christmas was viewed as not just a temporary pleasure, but also a powerful influence for stimulating the mind of the 'idiot'.

In 1910 Boxing Day was taken up with football and country walks. At 8pm 123 male residents gathered for a supper party hosted by Mr. Jarvis, the head attendant. The House Committee provided cold beef and plum pudding and each resident paid sixpence (2.5p), which paid for dessert. The patients then retired to the recreation hall for a concert programme that they had arranged themselves: consisting of songs, recitations, monologues and dialogues. Miss Hutchinson, the assistant governess, provided piano accompaniment.

The modern world reached Earlswood in 1970 when Santa Claus arrived at the Hospital by helicopter. In 1971 the GPO employees at Croydon paid for gifts for 84 of the children, two presents each together with sweets. The also provided a fibreglass slide, a swing and a scrambling net. The gifts were presented by 'Santa' Jock Briant, the schools sports and games master.

However, the seventies saw another change with the Institution having to provide money to purchase presents for the residents. Up to that date there had been a reliance on gifts donated by newspapers and other organisations.

On the first Thursday of the New Year the Winter Entertainment was held. This was an occasion when the friends of the Asylum and the influential ranks of society joined the staff and residents of Earlswood to celebrate the festive season. The day followed a regular pattern. First all would assemble in the dining hall at Earlswood. At three o'clock the presents from the Christmas tree were distributed amongst the eager residents. There would then be concert or dance music played by the Asylum band. Tea would follow and the day would end with some form of entertainment, usually a play or farce in which the staff played the main roles with great enthusiasm, although patients often contributed.

In 1863 the Morning Star reported on the event. The evening ended with 'An incident in the life of Robinson Crusoe' in which a large number of residents were introduced. In 1865 there was a three act 'Charade' – Act 1 'Blue', Act 2 'Beard', Act 3 'Bluebeard'. This was followed by a burlesque, again on the story of Robinson Crusoe. In 1864 the Christmas and New Year celebration were combined as the Xmas tea had to be deferred due to illness amongst the residents. Tables stretched along the whole of the main corridor groaning with their burden of cake, bread and butter, oranges and sweets for all 360 residents.

In 1866 the Asylum received a gift of 'lanterns for dissolving views' together with a large assortment of slides. Messrs. Collard donated a grand pianoforte. The evening event commenced with a Prologue given by the doctor. There then followed two plays, 'Jack the Giant Killer' and 'Bluebeard' performed by the officers and residents. The entertainment was repeated on the 18th of January for the family and friends. The hall and balcony was full to overflowing. Residents acted on the stage but were not in the audience. In 1868 the entertainment was a farce performed by the staff followed by a burlesque of Aladdin. The scenery had been painted by James Pullen, one of the first residents of the Asylum. The evening drew to a close at 10pm. On the 17th of January 1878 the entertainment took place in the covered gymnasium. J.B. Buckstone's farce 'Good for Nothing' was followed by Planche's extravaganza 'Sleeping Beauty', presented in seven tableaux. The scenery was produced by Mr. Wood, the schoolmaster, whilst the costumes were produced by Miss Godwin. In 1880 the demand for places at the evening entertainment was so high that it was necessary to put on three performances, all well attended.

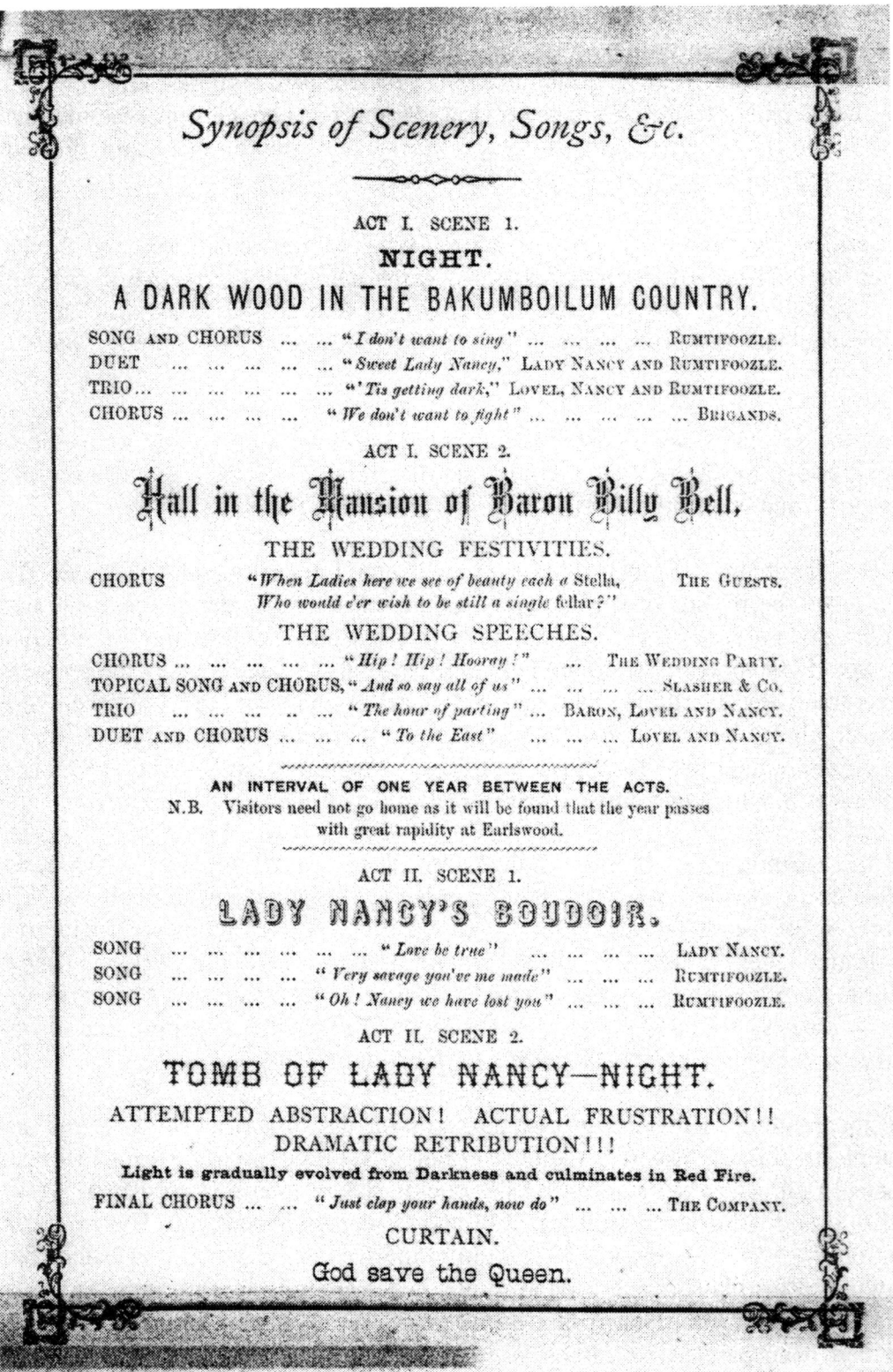

In 1883 the Entertainment took place on a Tuesday. Dr. Cobbold welcomed all the visitors. Mr. Ripley, the Chairman and Deputy Treasurer made a speech reporting on the death of Mr. Abbiss and the departure of Dr. Grabham who had left to become the superintendent of a lunatic asylum in New Zealand. Traditionally Mr. Abbiss had distributed tobacco amongst the attendants and, in his absence, Mr. Berry undertook this task. Gifts of toys and books, together with New Year cards, were given to all residents, many donated by friends after active canvassing by Mr. Nicholas. Then a huge basket of oranges was distributed by Mr. Kelsey. Tea followed, with fancy caps awarded as prizes. The friends of the residents provided an ample supply of crackers. The Asylum band played under the leadership of Mr. J. Franklin. There was a theatrical entertainment; a farce in 2 acts 'The Illustrious Stranger' or 'Married and Buried'. The programs were a work of art, produced by Mr. Street, the master printer at the Asylum.

In 1906 the *'Surrey Mirror and County Post'* made the following comment:

> **"On this occasion, as in previous years, staff and patients partook of the meal together and it was interesting to note the sympathy and tact displayed on the one side and the trust and affection evidently felt by the patients for their guardians."**

In 1907 the entertainment in the evening was the 'Society Pierrots'. In 1910 the patients' band, formed only twelve weeks before, performed in public for the first time. The day before the Entertainment the Asylum was open for friends and subscribers to visit and see the benefits of the system. Gifts received included several boxes of oranges, boxes of muscatels and money. The annual distribution of prizes occurred and the evening entertainment was provided by the 'Earlswood Minstrels'.

In 1912 the public distribution of prizes had to be called off because of an outbreak of scarlatina. However, the children did not suffer as they received their gifts in the schoolrooms. Tea was then held in the large dining room. All reportedly enjoyed the evening entertainment again provided by the Earlswood Minstrels.

For many years the toys were donated by the editor of *'Truth'* magazine for distribution at the New Year Entertainment. However this stopped in 1914 and the presents were provided by the Board instead. In 1920 the editor of *'Truth'* provided one third of the presents with the Board providing the remainder. In 1927 the Chairman of the Board presented the Institution with 'moving picture apparatus' and film shows became a regular entertainment for the residents. In 1984 *'The Sportman Club'* donated £100-150 for the purchase of one large present.

By 1970 the Winter Entertainment Day was an annual public meeting linked with a celebration of the foundation of the Institution. It was held on a Saturday to allow more relatives to attend. The guests were the family and friends of the residents rather than, as in the past, the leading members of society. An address was given and then the visitors toured the wards and other areas in the hospital. These areas were normally not open to the families and friends. It was normal practice for all meetings with relatives to take place in the visitors' room. There was also an exhibition of life at the Asylum. In 1975 the meeting commenced with three traditional songs. The address was followed by a Grand Skittles Match, with the 'Visitors' team being soundly defeated by the 'Residents'.

The Rebuild.

It is possible that the Board's insistence that the building contractor be held to the tender price was the factor that was to lead to future trouble. Whatever the reason, subsidence was noted in the west wing in October 1903. Then the walls of the tower appeared to be bulging. Investigation showed that the building had been constructed without foundations, simply 'floated' on the clay subsoil. The walls were cracking and being forced out by the roof, which

135

had not been tied in. The walls consisted of brick faced with thin blocks of stone. The stone used to face the building, quarried at Gatton on the outskirts of Reigate, was very soft and prone to flake. By the early 1900s the walls were already showing signs of distress. However, not only was the outside of the stone flaking but it was also separating from the brick core.

Early assessments estimated that an outlay of £30,000 would be necessary to prevent disaster. Appeals were launched, securities sold and loans were taken out. A total of £20,000 was raised but, despite strict economy, this was sufficient for only two-thirds of the immediate work. On the 17th of November 1904 *'The Daily Graphic'* carried an article entitled *'A TOTTERING ASYLUM. APPEAL FOR A NOBLE INSTITUTION.'* This contained the following information,

> **'Large portions of the building are, however, still unfit for occupation, some in a highly dangerous condition, and yet in a few weeks' time our whole available means will have been exhausted, and the work must be stopped, unless help is forthcoming. Are there none among the benevolent and wealthy who will step forward at such a juncture? Earlswood Asylum, the pioneer national institution for the care of this forlorn and helpless class, has for more than half a century conferred its priceless benefits upon thousands of inmates and their families. Its patron is His Majesty the King.'**

By July 1905 work was costing £1,000 per week. Never willing to miss a sporting opportunity, a cricket match was arranged between the Asylum and the special building team. Earlswood scored 126 runs with the opposition managing 39 in the first innings and 48 in the second, all before tea at 5o'clock. The match was scheduled to last until 7pm so after tea there was a return match that Earlswood won 84 declared, with the opposition 51 all out.

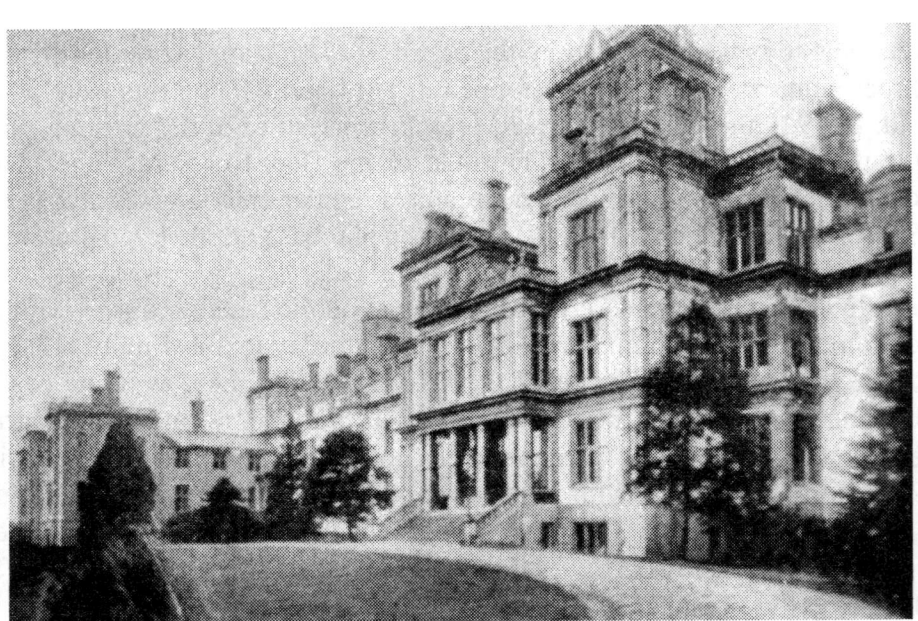

Earlswood – the original stonework

In September 1905 the *'Christian World'* reported that Earlswood was near the end of the restoration. In fact, it was only the first stage in a process that was to last nearly three decades. Large parts of the building had to be demolished and rebuilt. The northeast portion needed the most urgent work, the dining room and kitchen block required extensive reconstruction. The laundry and workshop block was also in need of prompt action. In the main building the northeast wing, the southeast wing and the two central staircases had to be shored up to prevent collapse. All the staircases needed to be replaced due to bad design. This would cost £22,000 of which £8,000 had been collected, £5,000 had been advanced on the mortgage and the remainder was outstanding. Walls had to be demolished and rebuilt either because of defects or to provide a base for steel trusses to support the roof. However, once urgent safety work was completed, the Board took the decision that the rebuilding would only proceed as money became available. The King donated 25 guineas towards the work.

By January 1906 most of the six fire escape staircases had been completed. The walls were underpinned to a depth of five feet. A water softener scheme and filter beds were in the process of being installed. However, £20,000-30,000 was still required to complete the works. All financial reserves were exhausted and 24 acres of land, previously mortgaged, had to be sold. The disruption to the life of the Asylum was tremendous but the medical superintendent and his staff were congratulated on how they had managed affairs.

In 1906 the southwest block was found to need work to the value of £2,500. The Charity had only £1,000 in hand. Board member Mr. William Hartmann, JP for Milburn, Esher, offered £500 if two other people would pledge the same. The offer was publicised in Surrey Mirror in August. By October sufficient funding had been obtained and work was underway. By this time the total cost of the rebuild had risen to £55,000-60,000. The Hospital, built to accommodate 600, could only accept about 450 patients because of the problems with the building. The media pointed out the plight of the Asylum and, therefore, the plight of the learning disabled population. 'The World' on the 12th of June 1906 made the following observation:

> **"It seems unnecessary and absurd that the London County Council should be proposing to waste a million or two upon a gorgeous house of assembly while the far more useful building at Earlswood is in need of the wherewithal to save it from becoming uninhabitable. The contrast almost suggests the advisability of erecting a joint domicile for the two institutions."**

In 1907 it became a priority to rebuild the east wing. A special fund was launched to raise the £25,000 necessary for the ongoing work. Mr. Hull, the Chairman of the Board, contributed £500 towards the total of £2,882 pledged at the annual festival dinner in May. In June a further appeal was launched for £6,000 to undertake work on the northeast wing. The King contributed 50 guineas, his second donation in two years.

In 1908 fund raising continued to complete a restoration of the northeast block. One hundred and twenty persons with epilepsy were housed in this wing. No residents were evacuated from the Asylum during the rebuild but for safety sake 40-50 of the patients were moved into a temporary building at the rear of the asylum, described by the 'Surrey Mirror' as "a commodious iron building"! Over the following two years the wards were restored. A new sanitation block was constructed for the males, comparable to that erected in 1901 for females. A spacious balcony was added for the open-air treatment of tuberculosis.

In 1909 a further appeal for £6,000 was launched. By this time donation rates were beginning to fall. By April only half the sum had been raised and a loan of £4,000 had to be taken out with the banks. In November a special court was held to authorise the use of more than the normal proportion of legacies, the rule being that 25% of the first £5,000 and anything above that figure should be invested. Certain investments also had to be realised.

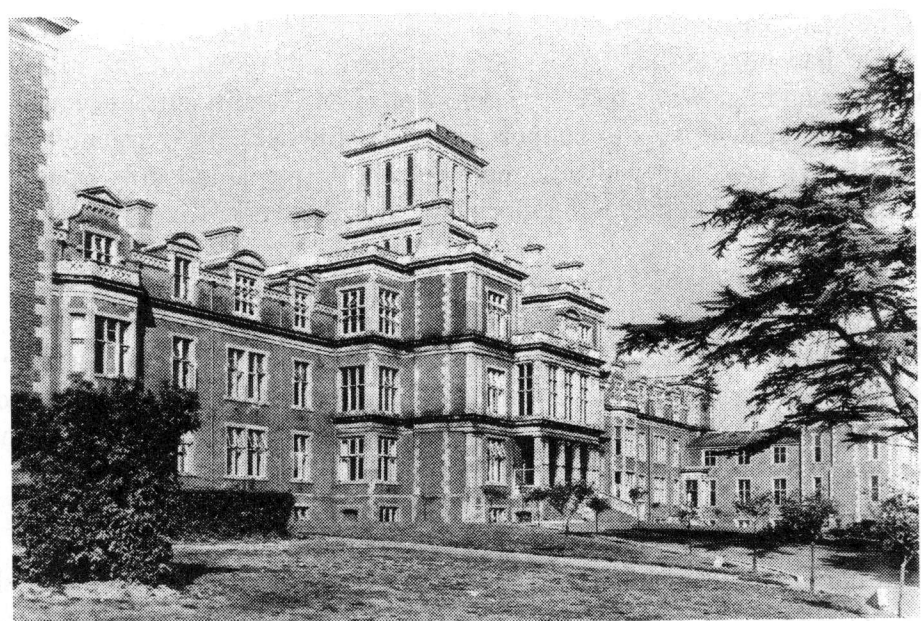

Royal Earlswood – after the rebuild

In mid 1910 the northeast wing was completed. At this point all work stopped. To date, £53,000 had been spent on the rebuild and £30,000 was still required. A method of treatment was found that negated the need to demolish and rebuild all the walls. Liquid cement was injected between the brick core and stone facing to 'glue' them together. Then red brick was used to reface the building to prevent further erosion. The character of the building was completely redefined. Only the workshop block was to retain its original gold coloured stone exterior. This method cost one tenth that of demolition and rebuilding, however, even this could not be immediately afforded.

In 1911 income increased slightly. In addition, £4,500 of securities were sold, together with a small piece of land, suitable for houses. The kitchen walls were successfully treated with the new liquid cement technique. Three thousand pounds were needed to similarly treat the laundry and workshop block. Unfortunately in November 1911 the kitchen ceiling collapsed suddenly and instant repairs had to be undertaken at an immediate cost of £250. In January 1912 the huge copingstones on the end of the laundry and workshop block were found to be in danger of falling. The entrance and roadway had to be blocked off and an emergency entrance arranged. Scaffolding was erected and the stones were removed.

The Charity made an appeal to all its subscribers requesting a special gift of ten shillings from each. By April 1912 only £700 had been received. The whole of the main block had been restored except for the rear central part comprising the dining room and the female epileptic ward. The kitchen was nearly complete. Earlswood was now £4,000 in debt. In May 1912 Mr. R. L. Hesketh FRIBA, the architect in charge of the restoration work retired and was replaced by Mr. W. Newton Dunn FRIBA. The work on the laundry and workshop block was still delayed by lack of funds. Every time the available money was close to sufficient it would be needed for some serious and urgent repair. The Workshop and Factories Act made it necessary for them to be inspected. The urgent need for modern laundry machines had been stressed. The kitchen and laundry equipment was in urgent need of replacement as routine refitting had been impossible in the face of the crisis with the building. The bill for kitchen equipment alone was in the region of £1,000. Every week the laundry processed 12,000-13,000 pieces and the equipment was worn out.

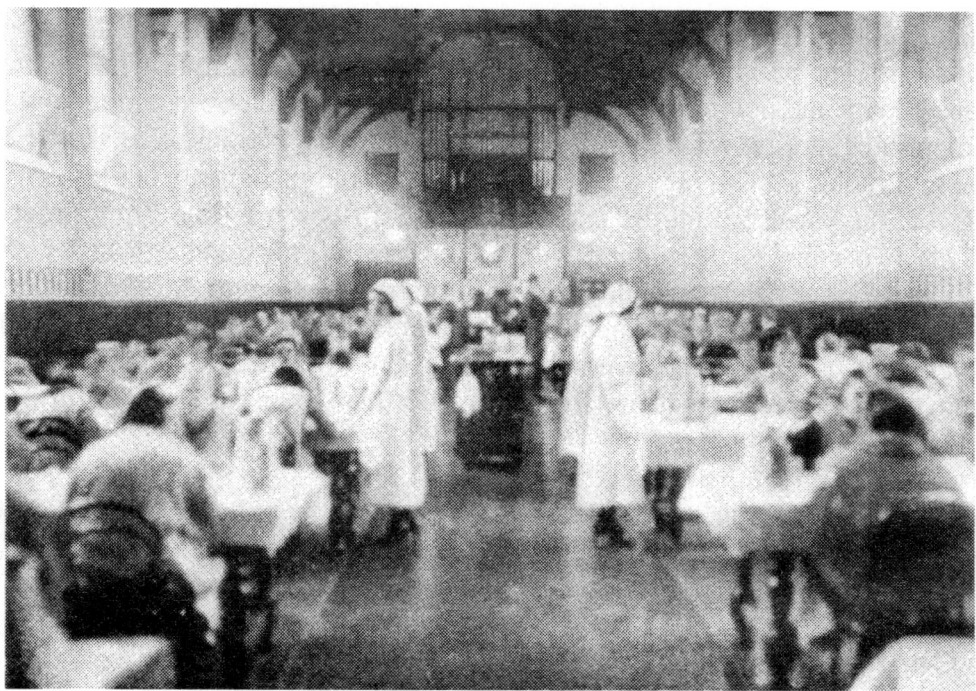

The dining hall

In 1913 the reconstruction of the two central staircases was a priority. This was not completed until 1915 at which time the water tank was also replaced having been condemned as unsafe. In August 1924 Mr. John Wright, engineer and clerk of works retired. He had worked originally for Ashwell and Nesbitt when they installed the steam heating, electric lighting and ventilation in the Institution. He then joined the staff at Earlswood for a period of twenty-five years during which time he oversaw the majority of the restoration program.

The rebuild of the laundry took place in 1926. One of the walls, the floor and roof were totally rebuilt and two walls were grouted. A Lyons steam disinfector was installed at the same time. The power had been previously supplied by a steam engine that had been in the Crystal Palace exhibition. This was now replaced. Throughout the whole of the restoration the laundry did not cease to function for a single day.

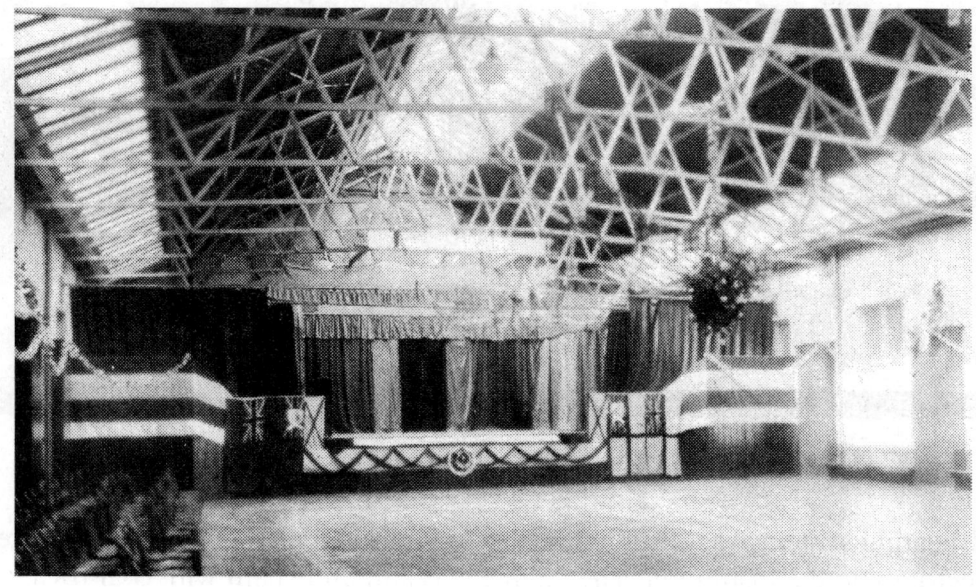

The covered exercise yard

The work still outstanding included the rebuilding of the workshops, the draining of land and the reconstruction of roads. The building work was undertaken one wall at a time. The area to be grouted was chipped down and pointed. The stone sailing course was removed and renewed in concrete, run in situ. The guttering was repaired and new rain water pipes installed. The end wall was demolished and replaced with nine-inch brickwork rendered in cement. The lavatory block roof was renewed, the party wall at the rear taken down a floor at a time. Iron girders were placed across the two main walls, topped with a concrete flat roof and finished with Ragusa covering. Concrete floors were installed down to the basement level. Modern toilets and washbasins were installed. This entire project was completed at a cost of £1,320. In April 1932 the *'Daily Telegraph'* reported that, with the restoration work nearly complete, the collapse of the foundation of three Lancashire Boilers would involve an outlay of a further £3,000.

The entire project eventually took nearly three decades. Ultimately, the building that had cost £29,400 to construct in the 1850s was to require over £80,000 for the restoration work.

The Twentieth Century.

From 1890 until 1899 Bridge House had been used as an isolation hospital. By 1900 it was being used to accommodate 16 male patients. In 1918 it was leased to E. E. Thompson for 21 years at £60 per annum, to include "messuage, dwelling house, coachhouse, stable/garage and garden". However, this arrangement was obviously discontinued early as reportedly by 1924 Bridge House contained the girls' continuation school.

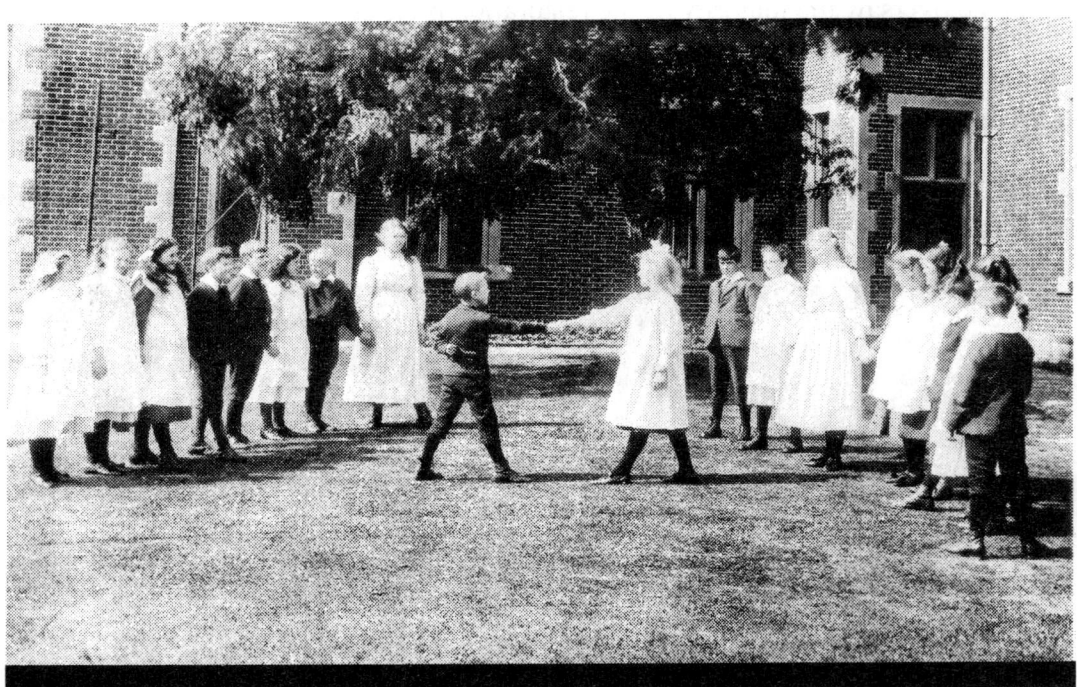

Learning etiquette

A central heating system was installed in the Asylum in 1910, together with a generator to supply electricity to the Institution. The regime was still quite hard with coal fires to heat most of the rooms and cold water for washing. Until 1934 the sexes were strictly segregated, even the staff.

140

Reigate Rural District Council.

ISOLATION HOSPITAL,

EARLSWOOD.

DIETARY ✠ TABLES

Adopted at a Meeting of the Council held on the 10th day of October, 1900.

ADULTS.	CHILDREN.
1.	**2.**
Enteric. Milk, Two Pints and a Half. Bread, Eight Ounces. Ice.	Milk, Two Pints and Half. Bread, Eight Ounces. Ice.
3.	**4.**
Scarlet Fever, etc. Milk, Two Pints and Half. Beef Tea, One Pint. Two Eggs. Soda Water.	Milk, Two Pints and Half. Beef Tea, One Pint. Two Eggs. Soda Water.
5.	**6.**
Convalescent Diet. Milk, Two Pints and Half. Beef Tea, One Pint. Two Eggs. Soda Water. Pudding. Bread, Twelve Ounces. Butter, One Ounce and Half. Sugar, One Ounce. Tea, Half Ounce.	Milk, Two Pints and Half. Beef Tea, One Pint. Two Eggs. Soda Water. Pudding. Bread, Eight Ounces. Butter, One Ounce and Half.
7.	**8.**
Meat, General Wards. Meat, Six Ounces (Cooked, and without Bone). Potatoes, Eight Ounces. Bread, Twelve Ounces. Milk, One Pint. Two Eggs. Pudding. Tea, Half Ounce, or Cocoa, ¾ Ounce. Sugar, One Ounce. Butter, One Ounce and Half. Cheese, One Ounce.	Meat, Three Ounces (Cooked, and without Bone). Potatoes, Eight Ounces. Bread, Twelve Ounces. Milk, Two Pints and Half. One Egg. Pudding. Butter, One Ounce and Half.

NURSES' & SERVANTS' DIET.

Meat, Six Ounces (Cooked, and without Bone).
Potatoes, Eight Ounces.
Bread, Twelve Ounces.
Milk, One Pint.
Two Eggs or Bacon, 1 lb. weekly.
Pudding.
Tea, Half Ounce, Coffee or Cocoa, ¾ Ounce.
Sugar, Two Ounces.
Butter, Two Ounces, or Treacle.
Cheese, One Ounce.
Beer, One Quart a day.

DIRECTIONS FOR SUPERINTENDENT.

BEEF TEA.—1-lb. of lean Meat, without Bone, to the Pint.
STRONG BEEF TEA.—2-lbs. of lean Meat, without bone, to the Pint.
CHICKEN BROTH.—One Chicken to each Pint.
ONE FOWL, 2-lbs., for Three Persons.
MUTTON —Leg and Shoulder.
BEEF.—Fresh.
RICE PUDDING.—One Ounce Rice, Quarter Pint Milk, Half Ounce Sugar, One Egg for Two Puddings.
CUSTARD.—Two Eggs, Half Pint Milk, Half Ounce Sugar.

Handscomb & Co., Printers, Redhill.

Isolation hospital menu

In 1932 the Institution took a 21year lease on the second floor of 14 and 16 Ludgate Hill at £300 per annum for use as the London office. In 1937 Earlswood had an electricity plant installed that provided sufficient electricity for the whole Institution and this was to serve the

Hospital until 1960. The steam engine and generator was built by Bellis and Morcom and could provide 20kilowatts at 700 r.p.m. In addition a complete system of telephones, fire alarms and electric bells was installed. In 1938 a new washing machine and airing room were installed in the laundry. A chlorination plant was installed on the brook water supply. Two new cottages were built for staff. In 1939 a new floor was installed in the patient billiard room. A further new washing machine was installed in 1941 and two other machines were overhauled. The parapet walls were repaired and the brickwork re-pointed on the west side of the infirmary building. In 1943 the outside walls of the main Hospital were re-pointed and a new drain was laid under the workshop block to remove floodwater.

In 1945 the female staff dormitories were converted into 28 single rooms, reflecting the new standards of privacy expected by staff. The following year all of the female staff accommodation in the east wing was converted into single rooms. New facilities were planned, to provide bathrooms, a shampooing room, an ironing room, drying room and rest room. This was completed in 1949. In the kitchen a cold store was installed for meat, milk and fish. The hospital obtained 150 new bedside lockers providing more storage for individual possessions.

In 1947 the washrooms on Victoria ward and the main corridor were redesigned. Victoria corridor and the west corridor were redecorated, the first part of a major program to improve the general environment now that the restrictions and demands of the war were over. In the kitchen standards of food hygiene continued to improve with the installation of a refrigeration plant and vegetable store.

In 1950 a staff mess-room was converted to provide accommodation for the finance department of the hospital group. A portion of the annexe was re-fitted as a nurses' training school. The mixed sex school, housed in the west wing, provided education for 54 residential children and four day cases. In 1951 and 1952 extra bathroom facilities were provided for the female patients. The water softening and filtration plant, supplying the Hospital with its fresh water needs, was replaced. The following year the hot water system and the cold water supply to the workshop block were renewed. Meanwhile plans were afoot to increase the size of Earlswood from 800 to 1000 beds.

In 1952 a cold water storage tank room was constructed and a new laundry receiving bay was built. Further improvements were made to the laundry in the following year and several parts of the Hospital, including the kitchen block, were refaced with new brickwork. 1954 saw renovations to the main kitchen and a new servery and washing up unit was provided in the staff dining room. Hospital Block was renovated and decorated. Further equipment was provided for the children's playground. The organ in the main hall was restored.

In 1956 the front hall and Victoria corridor were redecorated. Two ward kitchens were modernised and a new sluice was built on a male ward. There was an excellent patients' shop. The principle gas main was replaced. A contract was agreed with Messrs. C. W. Gosling Ltd to provide further electric power installations in the main and workshop blocks at a cost of £8,486. Further work was carried out on the laundry including the installation of a new ironing machine costing £5,000. The farm buildings were rewired. Part of the estate was sold to Reigate Corporation for housing and six houses were guaranteed for staff use.

Mains electricity reached Earlswood in 1957. The laundry rewiring was completed. By this time, 18,000 items were being laundered every week. Further improvements were made to two of the bathroom blocks for female patients, bringing them up to a modern standard for the time.

The external fire staircases were overhauled or renewed as appropriate. The northern side of the estate, bordering on to Brambletye Park Road, was re-fenced.

Indoors the visitor's room was redesigned. It was here that friends and family would still meet their relative, as it was not permitted for visitors to enter the wards. Small kitchens were created in two of the male wards, with sinks and hot plates. This allowed snacks to be made for and by the patients for the first time. The backdrop of the stage was replaced with help from the Reigate School of Art.

By 1958 the rewiring of the Hospital was largely complete and the Hospital generator was finally relegated to providing the backup supply. At last televisions could be provided for the residents. A large sanitary block was modernised providing toilets, bathrooms and kitchen facilities for three of the female wards. Also developed was a new linen room and laundry staff mess-room. Construction of a staff hostel with accommodation for twenty nurses was completed in November. Some of the resident staff, including all of the student nurses, were accommodated there. It was not just the practical issues that were considered. In order to brighten the wards, more cut flowers were provided and pictures were obtained from the Picture Library Scheme of the Red Cross Society.

In 1959 the Regional Health Board approved the second staff hostel and a bungalow was built for the Matron's use. Later this was converted into two single units of accommodation. A new sanitary block and sluice room was constructed for the Infirmary to replace a very old one. A completely new unit, containing toilets, baths and washbasins, was built for the 1st class ward and a modernisation program began for the bathrooms on the male side to give 6th and 2nd classes their own self-contained facilities.

Further equipment was provided for the children's playground, including swings, a roundabout, an old car and a London Bus. By now most wards had been provided with television sets, relatives donated the majority of them and the Friends of the Hospital the remainder.

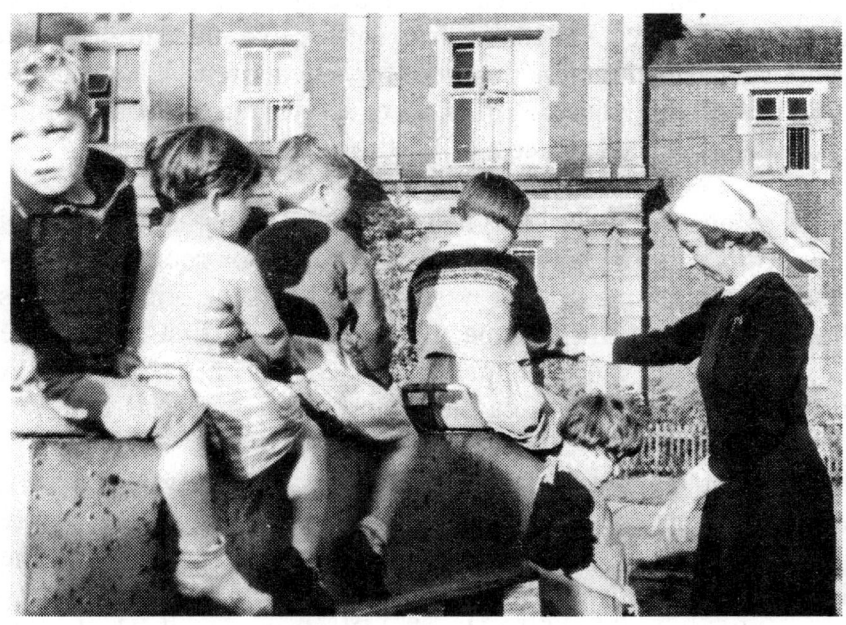

Playtime

The second hostel was opened in 1960, leaving very few staff resident in the main building. A third hostel was planned to complete the process of separating the staffs' home life from their work. The rooms vacated by the staff increased the space available for the patients. The male 4th class was reinstated and redecorated. A large dormitory on the male side was also renovated and the bathrooms modernised. The infirmary roof was renewed as a first stage in the buildings renovation program. In the laundry a new washing machine and a sock former were purchased.

Outside, a new roadway was constructed along the old Bridge House Road and an additional car park was built at the rear of the Hospital. London Transport donated a second bus for the children's playground. The buses continued to provide amusement for the children until they were eventually scrapped in 1966 and 1969. An enclosed area outside the nursery was surfaced and fitted with swings and a roundabout. The League of Friends provided funding for much of the equipment. In the front grounds a large shelter was provided for the use of the female patients, donated by parents, in memory of their daughter who had lived at Earlswood.

A staff social club was founded in 1951 and the building of a Staff Social Centre was commenced in May 1962. The Hon. W.S. Maclay C.B., O.B.E., M.D, performed the opening ceremony in October 1963. The King Edwards Hospital Fund provided £17,000 with the Regional Hospital Board providing £12,000 and the relatives and friends £1,000. In January 1967 agreement was reached to build an extension to the staff club, comprising two additional rooms and accommodation for the Hospital museum. The cost of approximately £8,000 was shared between the club and the Hospital with the King Edwards Hospital Fund for London providing a substantial sum towards the fitting out of the museum.

The first floor observation ward for females was completely revamped in 1961, the floors and ceilings were restored, the ward layout altered, the windows replaced and the wiring and plumbing renewed. The infirmary was also entirely refurbished. Early 1962 saw roof repairs on the main frontage. Improvements to the laundry included a collar and cuff press. A wheelchair store was erected for the male infirmary. New bathrooms were provided for the young boys' ward and the female epileptics' ward was redesigned.

The mid-1960s was a busy time with building on several sites. To the east of the Hospital construction began on the first two of four new villas, each to house 30 patients, and the new boiler house that would contain three oil fired boilers, with space for two more to be added later. At the other end of the site work began on a new school for 84 children. A new supply road had to be constructed together with over a quarter of a mile of service ducts. Phase I of the Earlswood redevelopment was complete in 1968 at a cost of £390,000.

The roof of the main building was repaired or replaced as necessary with re-slating and general weatherproofing. External stonework was renovated. All of the top floor rooms were re-plastered and decorated. A new internal phone system was installed and the King Edwards Hospital Fund provided funding for a patient lift. Pharmacy was re-sited on first floor of the infirmary block and enlarged to cope with the ever increasing demand on its services. A playground was created for the boy's ward. Several of the staff houses were modernised.

In 1966 the first phase of a planned development commenced with new offices, ward kitchens, better bathing facilities and new sanitary annexes for two of the bigger male wards. There were improvements to the Hospital Block; two staff houses were rebuilt, increasing the accommodation for married staff. In 1968 two female wards were reinstated, including reconstruction of sanitary annexes. Modernisation of the Hospital Block continued. The female Occupational Therapy unit was brought back into use. The staff club and museum were completed. The patients' shop was extended and modernised at a cost of £3,000, raised by the Friends of Royal Earlswood.

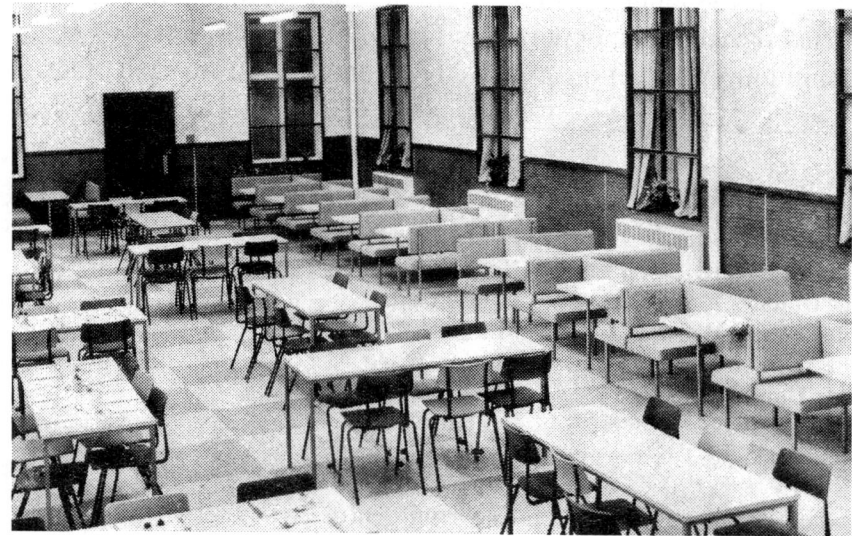

The self service cafeteria

In April 1969 construction of the second pair of villas commenced. The expected cost was £160,000 and the space vacated in the main building would allow extra room in the wards and accommodate the Nurse Education Centre. It was originally planned to build a further 13 villas in the mid-1970s for the cost of £708,000. All residents would then be relocated and the main building would be converted to house the service departments. However phases 3 and 4 were never completed as the idea of care in the community took hold.

In June 1969 a fire destroyed one of the female wards within the main Hospital, fortunately with no loss of life. The ward was back in use early in the following year. By 1970 the dining hall had been redecorated and was devoted to entertainment with music, cinema, concerts, carol singing and other seasonal events. 'Talkies' had replaced the silent movies of the past; westerns were especially popular apparently. The films were sent from a film library in London. Some residents preferred to watch the television instead.

Meals were now taken in the former recreation hall, a large light space behind the original dining hall. A cafeteria service operated giving the residents an opportunity to choose their meals and improve their everyday living skills by example. The residents were given training for six months before Viscount Addison of Stallingborough opened the self-service restaurant on the 25th of February 1970. Only the most disabled were to be fed on the wards. In 1977 a further fire damaged the museum and some of the exhibits.

Farming had ceased in the mid 1960s and the former farmhouse was converted into a hostel for men who were shortly to move into a community home, providing them with an opportunity to accustom themselves to a different style of life. The house had a sitting room, kitchen, office, and a room for the voluntary worker. Upstairs there were three small bedrooms and a bathroom. The Therapy Training Unit was re-housed in some of the farm buildings. Meanwhile, Bridge House became an occupational and social centre for mixed adult patients. Disposal of half of the estate was proposed but a decision was made that, for the time being, it should be leased.

In 1969 turnover of staff amounted to nearly 50%. In 1972-3 the new nurse education department was opened but there were concerns about the difficulty in recruiting adequate staff in an area of high prices and full employment. The new Art Therapy and Music Therapy departments were beginning to provide an opportunity for residents to express feelings, anxieties and dreams, even if they lacked language in the form of words or signs. In July 1973 the Gateway Club was inaugurated providing an opportunity for the residents of Earlswood and the Learning Disabled in the community to meet on an equal basis and learn from each other.

Units

Albert Ward	Henry Ward
Alexandra Ward	Hospital Block
Alice Unit	Louise Unit
Andrew Reed Ward	Margaret Ward
Anne Ward	Marina Ward
Brook House	Mary Ward
Charles Ward	Orchard Villa
Dutch Ward	Philip Ward
Edward Ward	Victoria Ward
Elizabeth Ward	Anderson Centre
Farm Villa	Bridge House
Garden Villa	Cozy Corner
George Ward	Parker Centre

Homes and units within Royal Earlswood.

From 1970 onwards, extra revenue allowed improvements in the residents' diet and meal service and increased the quality of clothing provided. The additional income also permitted better furnishings and decoration of the wards. Over the following two years the main building was completely rewired. Those residents displaced by the work were transferred to the Earlswood Home at Walton-on-the-Naze. In 1971-2 two further wards were reinstated, the fourth boiler was installed and conversion of the farm buildings began. In June 1984 five new gas boilers replaced the oil fired.

In late 1972 work began on the swimming pool housed in the old cattle shed, derelict since the end of farming at Earlswood. The design was based on the pool at Normansfield, 33 feet in length by 16 feet in width, two foot to four and a half feet deep. Heated to 75-85 degrees Fahrenheit, the water was filtered every two hours and there was a hoist to help the more disabled to enter and leave the water. Two-thirds of the funding for the project came from the King Edward Hospital Fund and the remainder from the 'Friends of the Swimming Pool'. In February 1969 Royal Earlswood had hosted a charity ball to raise funds for the pool and for toys for the children at 'Ellen Terry Home for the Blind and Subnormal'. The evening raised £1,100. The pool was opened on the 3rd of December 1973.

The Andrew Reed Unit was completed in 1973-4 as a residential facility for children. Elizabeth Home, where the younger children were housed, was divided into two separate units to provide a more homely environment. The remaining children of different ages and needs were housed on Phillip, Mark and Victoria Wards. Accommodation for a further 15 clients was provided by upgrading old staff quarters above the kitchens. There was considerable pressure on the accommodation for children. The Grange, a private Mental Health Nursing Home was contracted by the Regional Hospital Board to take children under seven years of age until space became available within the Hospital.

A new staff housing project was completed in 1975 and staff transferred out of the East and West Lodges. Work began on a three-year program to renew the Hospital heating system. The girls hostel was refurbished and the District Health Authority provided £4,000 for extra clothing. The enclosed area outside George Home was upgraded. The new residents social club was opened in February 1975. The building cost £8,000, the money coming from the Amenity Fund. The League of Friends paid for internal fittings costing £4,000.

The transfer of residents into the community began in earnest. Rehabilitation units, where residents could learn the necessary skills, were expanded. Matron's bungalow was converted to house four residents. Hostels outside the Hospital were created for clients as a half way house before they moved fully into the community. In 1973 a council house in Oxted was opened as Greengates Hostel. In 1977 houses in Dorking and Hurst Green were converted into further community homes for residents from Earlswood and Farmfield. In March 1978 Redstone Hall, a Social Service Nursing Home, was leased to East Surrey Health Authority and became a community home for residents moving out of Earlswood.

Alice	**20 beds**	**East Lodge**	**3 beds**
Redstone Hall	**11 beds**	**West Lodge**	**4 beds**
Brook House	**4-6 beds**	**Matrons Bungalow**	**4 beds**
Rusper Ward	**30 beds**	**Kiln Cottage**	**3 beds**

Rehabilitation units.

In the late 1970's a pioneer team at Royal Earlswood won a grant of £34,000 to launch a pilot scheme to provide special seating for six clients who, as a result of physical disability, could not be comfortably accommodated in normal wheelchairs. Earlswood farmhouse, recently vacated when the residents moved into the community, became the base for the Brook House Workshop, which provided specialist seating for those needing wheelchairs especially moulded to their shape. Furniture expert Petra Gormann and a consultant in rehabilitation, Dr. S. Jordan, based the chairs on the idea of 'shells' used at Chailey Heritage.

Earlswood, throughout its long existence, has always had a close association with the Royal Family. Queen Victoria was Patron of the Hospital, as was every monarch up to and including the present one. On the 28th of July 1981 the Hospital held a special Sports Day and on the following day there were outdoor parties to celebrate the wedding of Prince Charles and Lady Diana Spencer. Every resident was presented with a souvenir mug.

In November 1981 the Hospital rationalised its property holdings by disposing of 1 and 2 Leyland Cottages in Lonesome Lane, Reigate. The long planned third and fourth staff hostels were finally constructed. Woodfield and Great Meadow joined Garston Field and Six Acre Hostels.

In April 1982 work began on the extension to the staff canteen. Meanwhile conditions were deteriorating in the residents' cafeteria. In October 1983 it was decided that those on Charles Home would, in future, take their meals on the ward. Shortly afterwards the residents of Albert Home followed suit. This reduced the numbers using the cafeteria to 150 allowing the provision of a more homely environment. In February 1984 Ferguson Unit also ceased to use the cafeteria reducing the numbers further to 100. Final closure was discussed in October 1984 with the transfer of Edward, Alice and Alexandra residents back to their wards. In 1989 Royal Earlswood won the national 'Clean Catering Competition'.

At a cost of £120 per annum plus VAT Ruthworth and Dreaper tuned the organ, in the main hall. Watkins and Watson serviced the organ humidifier, at £46 per annum plus VAT.

Louise Unit, on the upper floor of the infirmary block, was established to provide respite for community clients whose parents and carers needed a break. Ellen Terry and Daffodil House were used to house children under 16 years of age who could no longer be cared for at home. In November 1983 plans were announced for the final ten children to be moved out of Earlswood into purpose built accommodation. Birchgrove and Beeches Bungalows provided a home for children with challenging behaviour and those frail children with high medical needs for the following 15 years. In 1987 Ellen Terry was developed as a community based short-term care unit with eight bedrooms before it was finally converted into a day unit for those with severe challenging behaviour.

A change of great significance occurred in August 1983. For the first time, a wardrobe was provided for each resident for the storage of his or her indoor and outdoor clothes. This became necessary as, for the first time, residents were to be provided with personalised clothing. Every resident was to be measured and fitted out with suitable clothes, in sufficient amounts, for their own needs and solely for their use. Prior to this residents simply drew on centralised clothes stores. In Victorian time, when family or friends wished to visit a resident at Earlswood they were required to give at least 48 hours notice 'so that clothes can be drawn from the wardrobe'. This method of providing garments had not changed for 130 years. This seems amazing to us now.

Another important change during the century was the degree of freedom given to the residents. For most of the century, if a resident desired to leave the Institution to visit, for example, an attraction in London, they would request leave and the Medical Superintendent would have the final say. However, it seems that the Medical Superintendent rarely saw the requests and that generally such outings were not permitted. By the 1970s such requests could be dealt with at ward level and would be granted if the resident was felt to be sufficiently able. Even late leave could be granted. Whereas it had been viewed as essential for staff to accompany residents on outings in the past, such an escort became difficult to provide due to of staff shortages.

Asylum staff after 1900

In March 1902 the Board passed a resolution in which it requested that Dr. Caldecott, the medical superintendent, and Harry Howard, the secretary should "make a thorough investigation of the system of the expenditure and financial management of the entire institution…"

The resulting report, presented to the Board on December 3rd, gives details of some of the staff employed by the charity in 1902. In the laundry there were 14 outside staff each paid two shillings and sixpence (12.5p) per day. In addition there were 12 indoor staff including the head laundress. It records that 12,000 items were washed every week including clothes and household linens. The hospital employed 16 needlewomen. The report stated that between them they cut out 2213 articles, made up 1515 garments including neckties and feeders, perhaps 'bibs', altered 92 garments and repaired 2144 items, including 1084 stockings and socks and all at a cost of £337. There were three linen room maids, five maids to work in the boys' wardrobe and three in the girls' wardrobe. At this time the residents of Earlswood did not

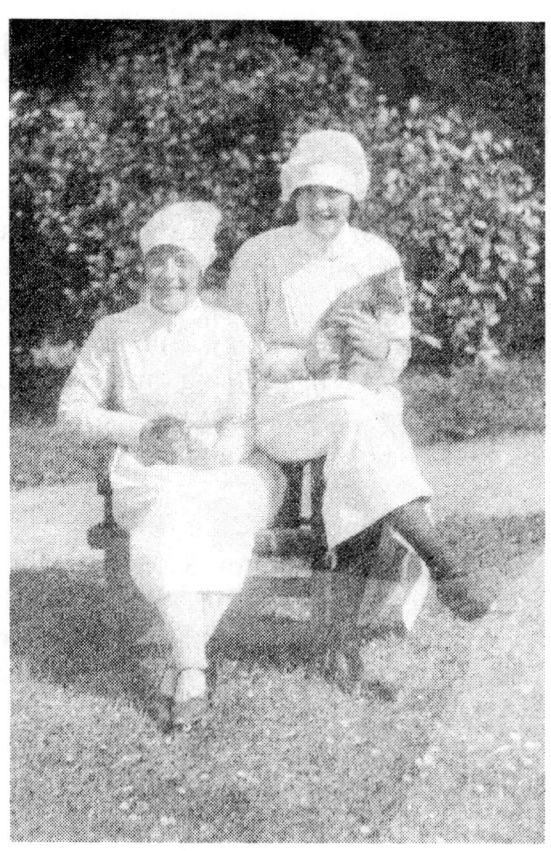

Nurses

have their own clothes but were supplied with clothes for everyday or Sunday wear from a central supply of garments. This prevented wastage as the children grew out of their clothes.

The report also detailed 33 nurses including the head nurse and night nurses. There were 50 attendants to look after the male residents, including shop attendants and the head attendant. There were some married women working on the male side. Four of the attendants provided one to one care for four private patients, a further two attendants each cared for two private patients and two staff were employed as relief for when the above were off duty. Class attendants staffed the 2nd, 5th, 6th and 7th classes. Trade attendants supervised in the various workshops, printers, tailors, boot makers, carpentry, mat makers, plumbers and painters. The staff who had some trade skills were paid a premium of five pounds a year. A master artisan, who was not of attendant status and lived outside the institution, oversaw each shop. His role was to supervise and train. There was also an attendant in the brush and basket shops, the farm garden and the kitchen. The remaining 'ordinary' attendants were known as housemen. During training times the ordinary attendants were employed with housework on the male side and some, under the direction of the matron worked on the female side.

Those with musical talent were still welcome amongst the employees of Earlswood. There was an excellent attendants' band and the performance time was the equivalent of one whole time attendant post. There were four staff in the engine shop and boiler room and ten people worked in the catering and stores departments. Each member of staff would have every other Sunday off duty.

In January 1907 the Surrey Mirror records the Winter Entertainment. It mentions that the instruction of shop masters and the management of the farm and gardens were under the care of Mr. Wells. The storekeeper was Mr. Taylor who was also conductor of the Asylum band. Mr. F. Nice was the hospital plumber. The head engineer and clerk of work was Mr. Wright and the matron was Mrs. Noble. Mr. Hull was Chairman of the Board. Other staff employed within the Asylum in the early years of the twentieth century included Miss Warmsley as Head Governess, Mr. Small was still Head Schoolmaster and Mrs. Scrivens was the Manager of the Holiday Home at Walton on the Naze.

In 1910 the 'Charity Record' noted that fifty percent of the staff at Earlswood had been employed there for 5 or more years, by 1912 this had increased to 57%. Only eighteen percent had been in the employ of the Asylum for less than a year. During the day there was one member of staff for every six residents, whilst seven staff were employed on night duty to care for the 460 patients. The top floor over the kitchens housed the nursing quarters at this time. There was a sitting room with a fire in it over the 4th class. The staff were able to purchase specially priced tickets on the railway, two shillings (10 pence) for a return ticket to London. Visitors received the same concession.

The regimen was quite strict, no nurse would be allowed to go out on Saturday night, Redhill being considered as an unsuitable place for a respectable woman. On other nights the doors were locked at 10pm and if a nurse were locked out on two occasions it would result in dismissal. The curfew was extended after the war to 10.30pm and in 1948, when the National Health Service took over, to 1.30am.

In 1914 Miss Warmsley, Mr. Wells, Mr. Wright and Mrs. Scrivens continued in their roles as head governess, farm manager, head engineer and manager of the holiday home respectively. Mr. Walker had taken the position of headmaster. Mr. Barnett conducted the male patient band and Mr. Taylor was listed as religious instructor, though whether this was the same man as that who was head store man is unclear. The head nurse was Miss. Hicks and Mr. Jarvis was head attendant. Many of the nursing and attendant staff had received no formal training, common sense was seen as the best preparation for the caring role. Married couples were put in charge of wards to create a more home like environment. In 1913 their combined wage was £52 plus board, lodging and laundry. One of the staff wrote that the food was good, with regular joints of meat. There were three staff employed in the male infirmary. Some of the patients helped with setting tables, washing up and making the beds.

During World War I the Asylum hoped to employ women to replace some of the men who had gone into the armed forces. However, the employment opportunities, and probably the wages, offered by the munitions factory in Salfords proved more attractive. When conscription was introduced Earlswood applied for exemption for its male staff. They were required to join the volunteers. They worked from 6am to 8pm six days a week and were expected to turn out for drill and fire watching. The Medical Superintendent was reputedly afraid of fire within the Institution, a real possibility given the new weapons used by Germany during the war. The Asylum had its own fire brigade and there were regular timed evacuations.

In 1918 the head attendant, Percy Worth got up a concert party called 'The Optimists'. They gave regular performances for the residents. Every Wednesday afternoon the attendants' band played in the dining hall, one afternoon for practice and one for a proper concert.

By 1920 Mrs. Noble had been matron for 33 years and Miss Warmsley had been head governess for 32 years. Miss Gear and Mrs. Mabel Yearsley replaced them in that year. Mr. Jarvis had been at Earlswood for 44 years, 28 as head attendant. Richard Smewin, who had been his deputy throughout, replaced him. The new mental health nurse training was introduced at Earlswood.

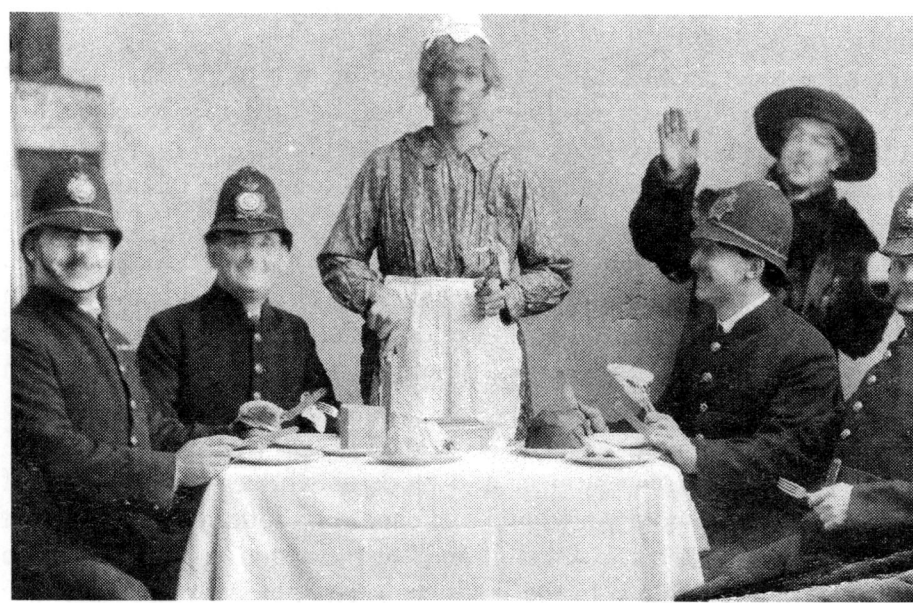

The Earlswood Optimists

A young man, Mr. Padwick, wrote about his appointment and early days at Earlswood in the 1920's. He applied to the hospital for the post of attendant and was invited to an interview with instruction to be prepared to stay. Obviously his interview by the medical superintendent was satisfactory as he was engaged for a period of three months probation. Taken immediately to one of the classes and placed under the supervision of the charge attendant Percy Robinson, he was instructed to feed two patients. During a quiet spell in the afternoon he was given permission to go to the post office and send a telegram to his parents to inform them of his successful appointment. He came off duty at eight in the evening and retired at 10pm to his room, accessed through a patients' dormitory. An eventful day for a young man.

He was woken at 6.30 the next morning and had to be on duty at 6.55am. There was no hot water and he records that shaving was 'done in the smoke room at any old time'. The patients were got up, washed and dressed and prepared for breakfast. In the staff mess there was a small loaf on each plate – this had to last all day. A lump of margarine, four ounces of cheese and 6oz of sugar were supplied, each on saucers, to last a week. The wall was lined with lockers nine inches square to hold the food. He was not impressed with the food, jam for Monday tea, marmalade on Wednesday and cake on Friday. The pay was fifteen shillings (75 pence) a week, paid monthly. If you played in the band you received an extra two shillings (10 pence) per week. The steward was also the bandmaster. He would advance money to new attendants until their first payday.

The attendants were allowed twelve days leave per year. This could be taken as a holiday, as full days, half days or quarters; the latter meant that you could finish at 5pm. No attendant was allowed out after 10pm unless he applied for late leave, which was not willingly given.

In November 1924 the death was announced of Mr. Hull, who had been Chairman of the Board for 27 years. A portrait was commissioned in his honour and contributions were sought from the other Board members and officers of the Charity. In December the Earl of Castlestewart agreed to take over as Treasurer and Chairman. The Vice Chairman was Mr. R.C. Grant, with Mr. Sydney Densham, who had joined in 1922, as Junior Vice Chairman. The following April Mr. H. Howard retired as Secretary, a position that he had held for fifty years. In recognition he received a gratuity of £500 and a pension at the rate of two-thirds of his £800 per annum salary.

Board members were often appointed because they brought with them some special skill, of use to the Institution. In February 1925 the Right Honourable Earl de la Warr was elected to provide expertise on farming. The constitution excluded women from positions on the Board. In 1923 they were allowed as honorary members with a maximum of four at any one time.

The Board met on the second Wednesday of the month at the London office for two hours. They attended a House Meeting at the Asylum on the first Thursday of the month from 11am to 1.30pm after which they had lunch before returning to London. The Medical Superintendent reported on matters of administration with the Farm Committee providing information on agricultural issues.

In August 1925 Mr. John Wright retired as engineer and clerk of works after 25 years of faithful service. He was presented with a gold watch and a cheque for £250, plus a pension of £126 per annum. He had originally worked for Ashwell and Nesbitt when they installed the steam heating, electric lighting and ventilation to the Institution. He then oversaw the entire rebuilding of the Asylum.

By 1927 the holiday home at Walton on the Naze was under the management of Miss. Bonnar and the farm bailiff was Mr. Horsburgh. In March 1929 the death was reported of Mr. Benjamin Densham, who had held a place on the Board for 25 years before his retirement in 1924. Mr. Densham had been responsible for the acquisition on the home at Walton on the Naze. In February 1929 Miss McMillan resigned as Matron. The post of Matron and Head Governess were combined and offered to Mrs. Yearsley at a salary of £230 per annum. In 1932 the Chairman of the Board, Mr. R.C. Henderson, passed away.

RULES FOR SERVANTS.

Charles Caldecott, M.B., B.S., Lond., M.R.C.S.,
Resident Physician and Superintendent.

1923

1 All Servants will be engaged on probation for three months, during which period one weeks notice on either side will be sufficient. Those who have been permanently appointed, and whose services may be discontinued, will be entitled to one months notice, or one months pay: and they will be expected to give the same notice, or to forfeit one months pay, in the event of their leaving the service before the expiration of such notice.

Servants who may be suspended from duty are not entitled to any pay or rations during the period of suspension.

Servants are liable to be summarily dismissed for misconduct, without notice or claim.

2 All Servants to wear the uniform of the Institution during the hours of duty. The males to wear the jacket or coat buttoned throughout. The females to wear their caps in the manner prescribed by the Matron. The hair to be worn plain and smooth.

The dress worn when out of uniform to be neat and appropriate, and subject to the discretion of the Superintendent or Matron.

No Servant to go out of the building without a hat or bonnet.

Each person must send his or her clothes, marked, to the laundry, accompanied by an inventory.

3 No communication is allowed between male and female Servants, except on the business of the Institution, during the hours of duty. No male Servant to go on the female side, and no female Servant to go on the male side, with-out permission from the Superintendent or Matron.

The female Servants are to use the extreme west staircase only, and the outer door to the left of the dining-hall. The male Servants are to use the extreme east staircase only, and the outer door to the right of the dining-hall. Standing and waiting at any time about the corridors, staircases, or entrance-doors is strictly prohibited.

4 The male Servants are not allowed to associate with the female Servants in the grounds

The female Servants will be permitted to take recreation in the grounds when off duty, but are to confine themselves to the paths and lower lawn at such times as the male Staff and male Patients are not there. When off duty for the day the female Servants will at once quit the premises or remain in the building. Servants are forbidden to enter the kitchen garden, farmyard, wilderness, or copse, and must not walk over the fields or meadows. Every female Servant having obtained a permit must at once quit the premises.

5 The private Nurses and Attendants are not allowed to have any other Servants in their rooms at any time without permission. No Servant is to make a sitting-room of his or her bedroom, nor to have a fire there without the sanction of the Superintendent. Smoking is permitted in the smoking-room only, and during off-duty hours.

6 No Servant is allowed to sing or whistle in the corridors or staircases. Bad language is strictly prohibited.

7 General Servants may read at breakfast and tea but not at dinner. Nurses and Attendants taking their meals with patients are not permitted to read at those times.

8 No Servants, except those authorized, are allowed to do cooking of any kind.

9 No Servants are allowed to pluck plants, flowers, or fruit of any kind, whether wild or cultivated, without the sanction of the Super-intendent, and they are required to restrict others, whether patients or Servants, from destroying and mutilating the flowers, shrubs, or trees of the estate. Birds' nests are not to be interfered with.

10 Servants not rising at the proper time in the morning will have a portion deducted from their leave of absence.

11 No Servant is allowed to send a patient beyond the grounds without permission.

12 No Servant is allowed to employ patients to draw water, or empty slops, without special permission from the Superintendent or Matron. No patient is to be allowed to dress or undress another, or to assist in doing so, except under the guidance and continuous observation of an Attendant or Nurse.

13 Servants are not allowed to post letters or execute commissions for the patients without permission. They are also forbidden to write or communicate in any way with the friends or relatives of an inmate.

14 No Servant is allowed to take charge of the money of patients, or to traffic with them in any way.

15 It is required that no servant shall see or know of any patient being unkindly treated in any way, without reporting the same to the Superintendent.

Neglect or ill-treatment of a patient is a misdemeanour, and may be punished with imprisonment for a lengthened period.

16 The leave of absence granted to Ser-vants is to be subject to the exigencies of the service of the Institution, and can never be demanded as a matter of right.

It is also liable to be partially or wholly withdrawn in the event of misconduct.

17 All members of the Staff are expected to make themselves acquainted with the Fire Rules, and must remember that in case of Fire the first thought must be the removal of the Inmates, who may be in danger, and next to give the Fire Alarm.

18 No Servant is allowed to enter a Public House when on duty.

19 No Alcoholic Stimulant of any kind is to be brought into the Institution without the previous sanction of the Superintendent.

20 All Accidents or Injuries to Patients should be immediately reported to the Head Nurse or Head Attendant.

21 All members of the Staff are requested to bear in mind the importance of setting an example to the Inmates, by keeping strict control over their temper, language, and conduct generally both at work and play, and when on and off duty, remembering that the 'Feeble-minded' are great imitators, and are much aided in controlling themselves by the upright and moral example of their superiors, and vice versa, are very prone to copy their vices.

By Order of the Board,
CHARLES CALDECOTT, M.B., B.S., Lond.,
M.R.C.S.,
Resident Medical Superintendent

Discipline was strict. Even as late as 1934 staff were segregated, it was forbidden for male and female staff to converse together, except in the line of duty. Notices were posted around the Hospital warning of grave consequences though these were not specified.

Until 1931 the head night attendant was George Flint. There is a record that in 1938 Miss Wade was managing the Earlswood Home. F Sargant was head attendant in 1939 and in 1942 the Chief Male Nurse was Mr. Wrake and the Printing Office shop-master was Mr. Frederick Hooker. A resident in 1942 described the male staff uniform, dark blue with a peaked cap, very distinctive when accompanying clients into the community. No resident was allowed out alone in those days.

Mr. Horsley resigned as farm manager in May 1941, to be replaced by Mr. Little. In 1942 Mr. Sydney Densham resigned due to ill health, he had been Chairman of the Board since 1933. In 1945 Mr. Jenkins retired after 46 years, most recently employed as clerk and steward. Mr. Harry Parker retired after 33 years as stoker. Efforts were afoot to improve the working life of the staff. It was decided that, as soon as staffing levels permitted, the five day week, so far only applicable to the male attendants, would be extended to the nurses. The shortage of nursing staff was to continue into the 1950s. In 1956, after a ballot of staff, the long day was replaced by a shift system.

The Annual Report for 1948/9 recorded the retirement of Mr. Tompkins after 37 years, many of which he spent as head school attendant in the boys continuation school. Also mentioned was the death of Percy Worth after 40 years of faithful service, ultimately as chief male nurse. Mr. H. Stephens retired in October 1950 after 46 years as secretary to the Hospital Management Committee. He was presented with a silver salver appropriately inscribed. Mrs. Stephens received a handbag. Bernard F. Thompson succeeded Mr. Stephens.

On the 30th of June 1951 Mrs. Mabel Yearsley retired from the post of head teacher and matron that she had held for twenty-two years. Miss B.M. Dover was appointed as matron and head of the training school, which currently had 23 student nurses. Meanwhile Miss J.E.B. Cunningham was appointed head teacher. Mr. E.L. Wrake was chief male nurse and Mr. and Mrs. A.R. Bowen managed the holiday home in Walton on the Naze, positions they still held in 1968. The farm manager was Mr. Knight. By 1956 he had been replaced by Mr. C.H. Morrall. In 1957 Mr. P.B. Waldron was senior clinical psychologist and Mr. H. Hall was chief pharmacist, the first full-time pharmacist having been appointed in 1956. In 1960 Miss E. Rushton was appointed as speech and language therapist. Her work was concentrated on children and groups were founded for boys and girls to work on vocabulary and articulation.

In 1959 Earlswood staff included 56 female nurses, 76 male nurses, two educational psychologists, a matron, a chief male nurse, and a large ancillary staff. In 1962 there were problems recruiting staff to replace the retiring speech and language therapist, occupational therapist, school supervisor, pharmacist and hospital engineer. In 1963 Mrs. M. Moore became school supervisor and J. Connolly, head tutor.

In 1967 Miss D.K Lee took over as chief pharmacist and Mr. Morrall became estates manager. In 1969 Mr. Waldron was Principal Psychologist and Mrs. D Cortazzi was Senior Psychologist. Mr. G Carter was catering manager. Mr. Connolly was Principal Nurse Tutor with Mrs. Connolly as Assistant Nurse Tutor. Mrs. V Hill was Director of Technical and Social Training. The Church of England Chaplain was Rev. Ruddock with the Free Church Chaplain Rev. Binney.

The staff employed consisted of 144 male nurses and 135 female. There were 25 male and 10 female student nurses. There were 198 males and 140 females employed in other capacities.

Staff turnover was high with almost half of them changing in a year. However, there were some long-term staff leaving too. Mr. Pearson, group engineer, and Mr. Homer, supplies officer, both left after 20 years service.

In 1969 the Hospital received a visit from the Secretary of State for Social Services, Richard Crossman, "to find out what makes it such a successful hospital for recruiting staff". Earlswood had one of the highest staff - patient ratios in any learning disability hospital in the country. He toured the hospital with Dr. David Anderson, physician superintendent, Mr. L. White the group secretary and Mr. T.E. Packer the chairman of the management committee, talking to the staff. He was impressed by the high morale.

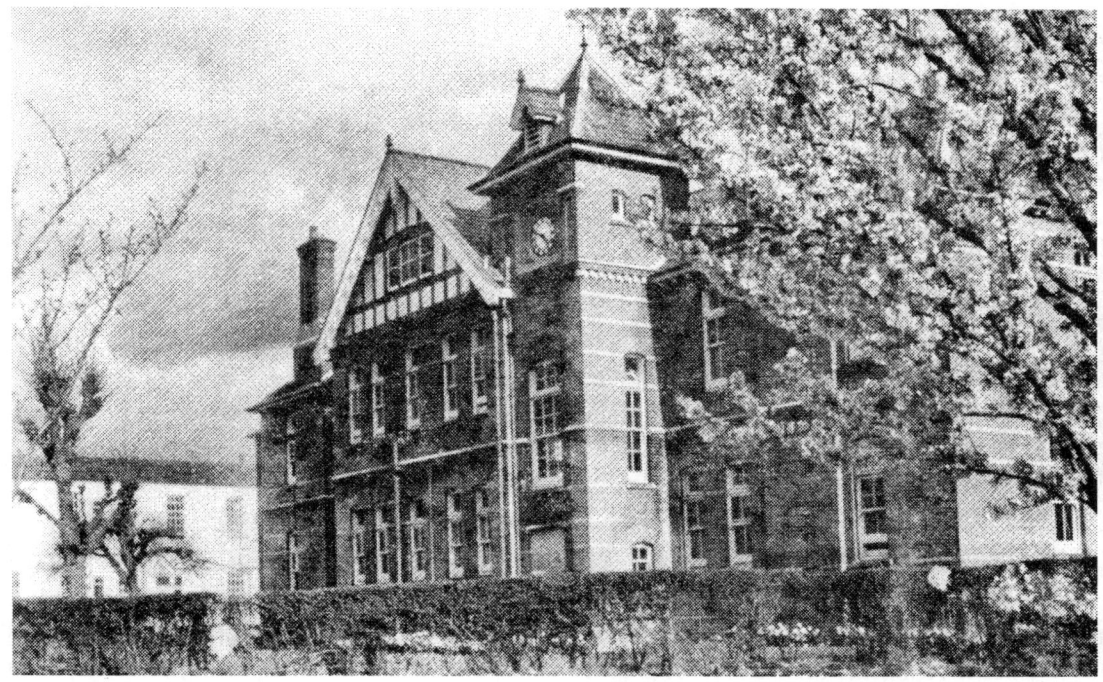

Forest Hospital

By the 1970's the staff of Earlswood included approximately 280 nurses, 50 therapists, 48 domestics, 20 catering, 20 administration, 5 engineers, 4 drivers, 12 porters, 14 wardrobe staff and 10 persons employed in the laundry. In 1971 the chief nursing officer was Mr. J Bowe and Dr. Livingstone had replaced Miss Lee. These staff cared for 500 residents. The first full-time social worker, Mrs. A.C. Crindrod, was appointed in 1973-4. Mrs. M.M. Arnaud was the hospital physiotherapist and Mrs. M. Thompson was speech and language therapist. Mr. E. Dinsdale replaced Dr. Livingstone as staff pharmacist.

In 1975 Mr. A.R. Cooper was appointed as Deputy Administrator following a career in the RAF, and Mr. R. Roberts commenced as Community Nursing Officer. Meanwhile, Mr. H Cliff Parry retired from his post of Medical Records Officer after 45 years, interrupted only by war service.

In 1979 there was a divisional nursing officer, Mr. J Bowe, two senior nursing officers and 8 nursing officers. There were 51 sisters and charge nurses. Royal Earlswood employed approximately 200 part and full time nurses, 50 professional and technical staff, 35 administration staff, 200 ancillary staff, 30 artisans and three chaplains.

Generally the staff were very happy but occasionally the hospital was troubled by the industrial unrest that was common in the country as a whole. On the 22nd of September 1982 there was a one day strike affecting the staff working in the catering, transport, laundry, portering, stores and wardrobe departments.

Farmfield

Following the creation of the National Health Service, Earlswood ceased to be a private institution and became part of the national provision. With two other hospitals, Forest Hospital

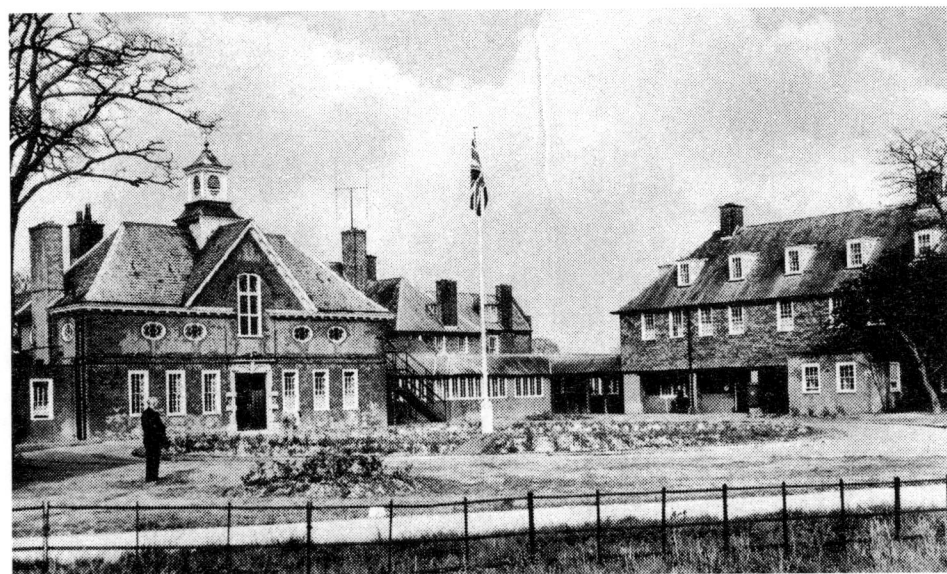

Farmfield

near Horsham in Sussex, and Farmfield, near Charlwood, it formed the Royal Earlswood Group. Forest Hospital left the Group in 1974 to become part of the Cuckfield and Crawley District under West Sussex Area Health Authority. Farmfield has continued its association with Learning Disability services in Surrey to this day.

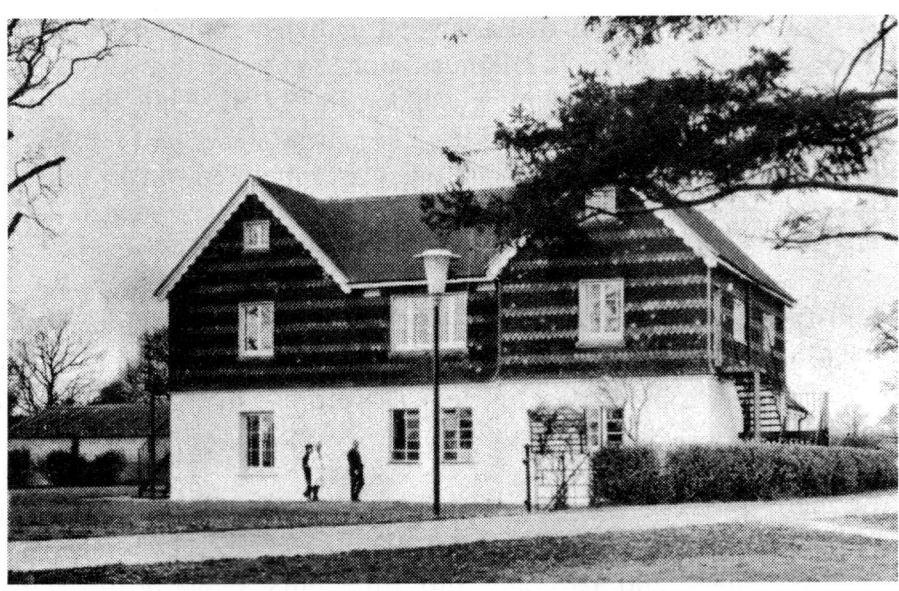

Farmfield

Opened in 1925, at its height Farmfield housed 180 men in five residential blocks. In 1969 the complete rebuilding of the former farm hostel resulted in premises that set the standard for a modern hospital. Known as Charlwood Ward, it was opened in December 1970. The other blocks were also named after local villages, Faygate, Ifield, Hookwood and Rusper. There were training facilities, a workshop, school, all purpose hall, also upgraded in 1969, and large outdoor recreation area. The outdoor Therapy Training Unit, which made concrete building and garden products in great quantities, had been re-housed in converted farm buildings.

```
374 Acres, Park, 12 Bed and Dressing Rms., 4 STALLS, COTTAGES.
SURREY (between Redhill and Three Bridges, only fifty minutes
From City and West End, 2 miles from station). - For Sale, an
exceptionally attractive small Sporting and Residential Freehold
ESTATE of about 374 ACRES, all lying well together in a ring fence,
and possessing considerable road frontage, with several sites on
rising ground, suitable for the erection of gentlemen's residences if
desired.
The sporting attractions are very considerable, the ground is good for
partridges, and the adjoining owners preserve. 108 brace of partridge
were killed in one day this season on the adjoining property.
The residence stands about 200 ft. above sea level, almost in the
centre of the estate, within a well-timbered park of about 100 Acres,
and is approached by a carriage drive nearly half-a-mile in length,
which winds through the park. The house is a quaint and picturesque
old structure and contains: tiled porch, square entrance hall 18 ft.
by 13 ft. 6 in. with dog grate, tiled fireplace and carved wood
mantel, morning room with square bay and casements, and opening to
conservatory, drawing room 20 ft. by 16 ft. with square bay and
casements opening to the lawns, capital dining room 27 ft. by 18 ft.
and 11 ft. high, with three casements opening to arched verandah,
marble mantel with tiled hearth, butler's pantry, store room,
servants' hall, kitchen and scullery with dairy, two larders, and boot
hole in the house yard; over the offices are three rooms for men, and
fruit store; on the upper floor are eight family bed and dressing
rooms, bathroom with hot and cold supplies, w.c., four attic bed
rooms, w.c., box room &c.; heated by hot water; outside are earth
closets for gentlemen and workmen. Water by force-pumps from well and
the Caterham
Company are laying mains close by. Stabling of three stalls and a
loose box, coach-house for three carriages, chaff-house, harness room,
and two rooms for men ovell timbered pleasure grounds, shady lawn,
tennis court, rose garden, ornamental lake and island, fed by springs,
boat-house, vinery with vines in bearing, capital walled kitchen
garden with greenhouse. Small brick-built farmery of two loose boxes,
cow-shed and piggery. The land has been highly farmed and well
drained, every pasture field being supplied with water; this is
recognised as the best farm in the parish. There is a capital
farmhouse containing large hall, dining and drawing rooms, six bed
rooms, three attics, dairy, kitchen, scullery, larder &c.; nag
stabling, and ample farm buildings with stack yards, &c.; also two
good cottages and small buildings. About 200 Acres are under grass, a
few small spinneys, and the remainder, easily worked arable land of
good quality. Telegraph office and church 11/2 miles.
The property is subject to a tithe of about £35 value in 1896; land
tax £2-11s-3d (£2.58). Rates and taxes very low. Price, including the
valuable timber, £15,000. The tenants' right, and usual tenant's
fixtures and fittings by valuation. The whole of the live and dead
farming stock can be purchased if desired. Personally inspected and
recommended.
N.B.- Would be let furnished.
```

Advert as it appeared in 1900.

The Farmfield estate had an interesting history before becoming a hospital for the Learning Disabled. In the mid 19th century it was owned by the Right Honourable William Pitt, Earl Amherst. He sold the property to W.J.J. Fish on the 22nd of October 1860. Following the death of Mr. Fish in 1882 the land was sold to the de 'Eyncourt family. There is a record that shortly

159

before 1900 a Lady Summerfield converted the farmhouse into a 'Home for Female Inebriates'. It is unclear who Lady Summerfield was as in 1900 the de 'Eyncourt family sold the land to London County Council. In 1901 villas were constructed and the property became a "state institution for difficult young adults who had passed through the London Courts". It was run as a home for those with serious drink problems and was know as the Farmfield Reformatory for Inebriates.

Records show that in 1910 there were 76 people resident there at a cost of £1-12s-3d (£1.61p) per week. After allowing for funding contributed by the treasury, the cost was £1-1s-7d (£1.08p) per week. The Reformatory had originally cost £44,013 and there was an outstanding debt of £36,540. The annual cost of the debt was £1,996. By 1912 it was felt that the Reformatory was no longer viable and the 'Public Control Committee' investigated the disposal of the property. However, at the time land values were low so it was decided not to sell.

By 1921 the buildings had fallen into disrepair. Following renovation the London County Council opened an institution for 'Mental Defectives' on the first of January 1925. This continued until 1948 when it was taken over by the National Health Service and became part of the Earlswood Group. Until 1955 it was a 'half-way' house for difficult cases, those who did not improve would be transferred to Rampton Hospital. It eventually became an open hospital for male patients with challenging behaviour.

A number of cottages were erected by the entrance to the estate and these provided accommodation for some of the staff. There was also two properties known as Kiln Cottage and Farmfield Lodge

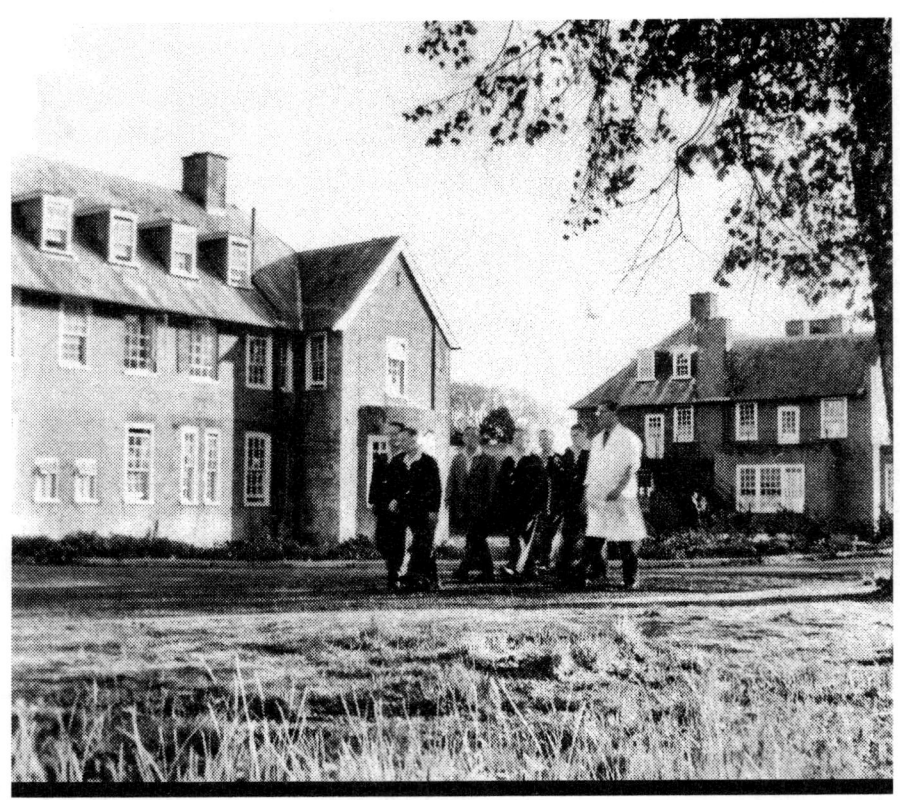

Life at Farmfield

Farmfield had 360 acres of land that was farmed until 1963, at which time some of the land was leased to a local farmer for grazing. In 1968 280 acres were sold at auction, the remainder was retained and 75 acres were leased. This generated £1,608 per year for the Hospital. The cricket and football fields were retained.

By 1987 Hookwood Ward had closed. The other four residential units remained together with an Occupational Therapy Department, WRVS shop, Social and Recreation Department, staff quarters and residents club. The residents were gradually transferred into the community or to Royal Earlswood and on the 18th of September 1989 Rusper Ward closed. On the first of October 1989 the flats at Shrewsbury Road, Redhill were ready for occupation by the remaining 18 residents of Farmfield. Open days were held on the 10th and 11th of October before the men moved into the new flats on the 21st and 22nd of October 1989. Charlwood Ward now closed, marking the end of Farmfield as an Institution.

Walton Hall.

The residents of Earlswood were luckier than many in Edwardian England in that they had regular holidays. Mr. Benjamin Densham, a member of the Earlswood Board, bought a house in Essex in 1904 which he leased to the Asylum. Originally Walton College, it was renamed 'The Earlswood Home', later Walton Hall, and was situated in Naze Park Road, Walton-on-the-Naze. It was intended to make the home self-financing and a permanent part of the Institution. Originally rented, the Charity hoped eventually to be able to buy the property. This it achieved in 1923. Initially, up to 25 residents could holiday at Walton at any one time.

The idea for the holiday home arose in 1897 when it was proposed that "the Diamond Jubilee of our beloved Queen" and the 50th anniversary of the Asylum, should be commemorated by establishing a permanent seaside home on the south coast. It would be used as a convalescent home for patients recovering from illness and as a place where paying cases could, "in carefully selected groups", benefit from a "sea-side change". In the event the home on the south coast was not to be established for a further ninety years. However, the home in Essex proved very successful.

The property comprised the following accommodation; on the ground floor three public rooms, a dining room, a billiard room, kitchen, scullery and larder, a toilet and 'ablution room'. On the first floor there were four dormitories, a single room in case of illness and three other bedrooms. In addition there was a bathroom with two baths and a basin, two toilets, a lobby linen closet and a landing. In the attic there were two further bedrooms. In addition to the house there were outbuildings, a boiler house, a small summerhouse, shelters and two and a half acres of ground, half an acre of which was enclosed within a wall and used as a kitchen garden. Lawns and a fruit garden surrounded the house. There were greenhouses, a potting shed and sheds for storage of garden tools.

In 1938 it was planned to increase the accommodation at the Home with the construction of a bungalow to house the Officer in Charge and his family. However, the war forced the abandonment of this plan and it was not re-instated until 1961.

During the war the holidays came to an end and the home was requisitioned by the Secretary of State for Air. The Charity was paid £202-8s (£202.40) including fire insurance of £2-8s (£2.40) per annum. The Home was de-requisitioned in 1945 but unfortunately lack of staff prevented it being reopened for several years. Reopened in 1947 it was closed again in mid 1948 for extensive repairs to be carried out. The Home eventually reopened in February 1950. Wireless sets were installed for the first time. During the year 134 patients from Earlswood, 28 from Farmfield and 32 from Forest Hospital enjoyed a holiday at the Home, in groups of 20. Those from Farmfield stayed a week whilst the residents from Earlswood enjoyed a stay of a fortnight. In 1952 television was provided and enjoyed by 170 visitors from Earlswood.

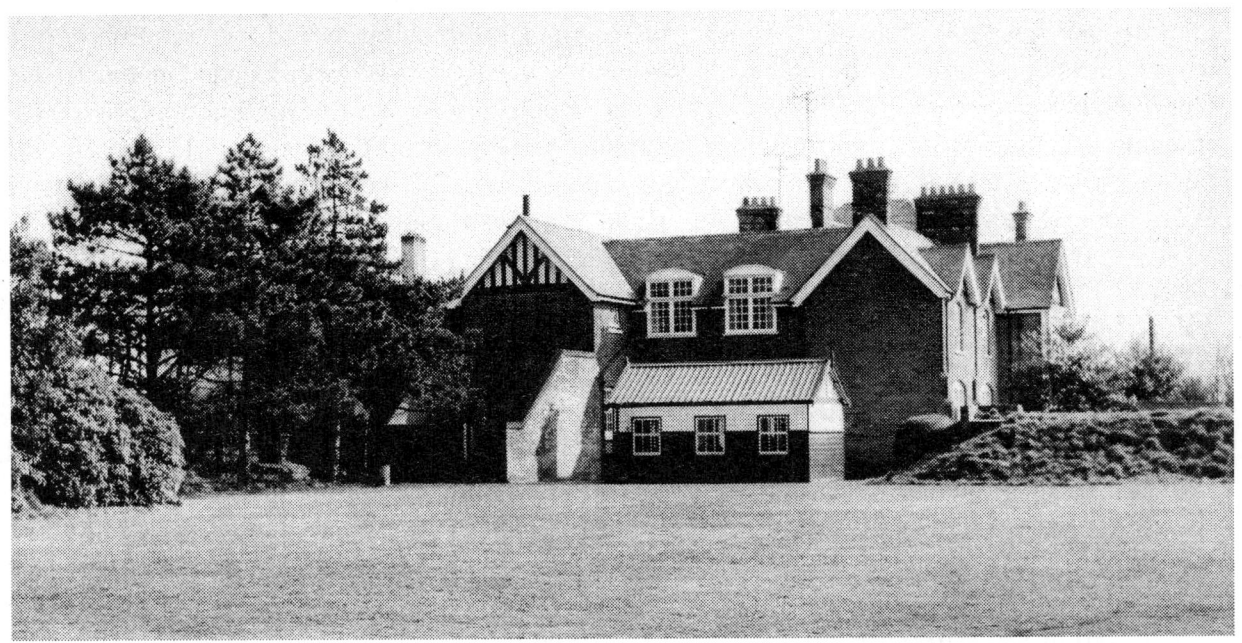

Walton Hall

The Home was regularly inspected by Hospital Visitors. Their record book survives from the early 1950s. In July 1950 they recorded the presence of seven holiday-makers. They were pleased with the improvement in the general appearance of the Home although they noted that the outside was in need of a coat of paint. They were pleased to record that the residents received a good supply of fresh vegetables provided by Mr. Balls the gardener. The Home closed for six weeks at the end of the summer to allow for staff holidays. The next visit was in November when the residents were ten 'working boys', all over 16 years of age. They stayed over the winter to help with painting the outside of the Home. They visited the cinema twice a week and had occasional outings by car. Each week they received between 1/6 (7.5p) and 6/- (30p) as pocket money.

Those on holiday received money from their family or would be given 6/- (30p) by the Hospital. They brought with them three changes of underwear. Sheets were kept at the Home and the laundry was sent to Earlswood. The diet was full and varied with breakfast, a cooked lunch, a high tea and cocoa and sandwiches at 8pm. Residents were weighed weekly. The Officer in Charge was Mr. Bowen and his wife who were both nurses. In addition there were two housemaids, a resident cook and a gardener. Two nurses accompanied the clients from Earlswood. The local G.P. provided for the health of those at the Home.

In 1953 two beach huts were provided for the holidaymakers at the suggestion of the Hospital Visitors. One was used for making tea and the other for drying bathing clothes. A swing settee was placed in the garden. In 1955 fire exits and smoke detectors were installed on the second floor allowing these to be used for patients. A small library was available. In 1960 a replacement boiler was installed.

162

It was common in the 1950s and 1960s for a party of male patients to stay at Walton Hall from January until March to help with the garden and repairs to the house. The Home was then available for holidays from April until November. In 1969 the central heating was replaced making it more comfortable for those taking an early or late holiday. The weekly cost of maintaining a client at Walton Hall was recorded in 1969 as £12-14s-8d (£14-73), nearly £3 less than the cost of living at Earlswood Asylum. By the following year it had risen to £16-3s-5d (£16.17) whilst the cost at the main Asylum was £17.46. This increase may have reflected a reduced number of clients accommodated at Walton Hall in 1970 as by 1971 costs had fallen to £13.41 per resident per week. During this time numbers were maximised as the Home was utilised to accommodated Earlswood residents displaced during the re-wiring of the main Hospital building. In 1973 the weekly cost was £18.78.

In 1975 work began on a ground floor extension. The new dormitory allowed wheelchair bound patients to enjoy the benefits offered by the holiday home. The cost of the development was £5,700. The target was that every patient at Earlswood should have at least one weeks holiday a year.

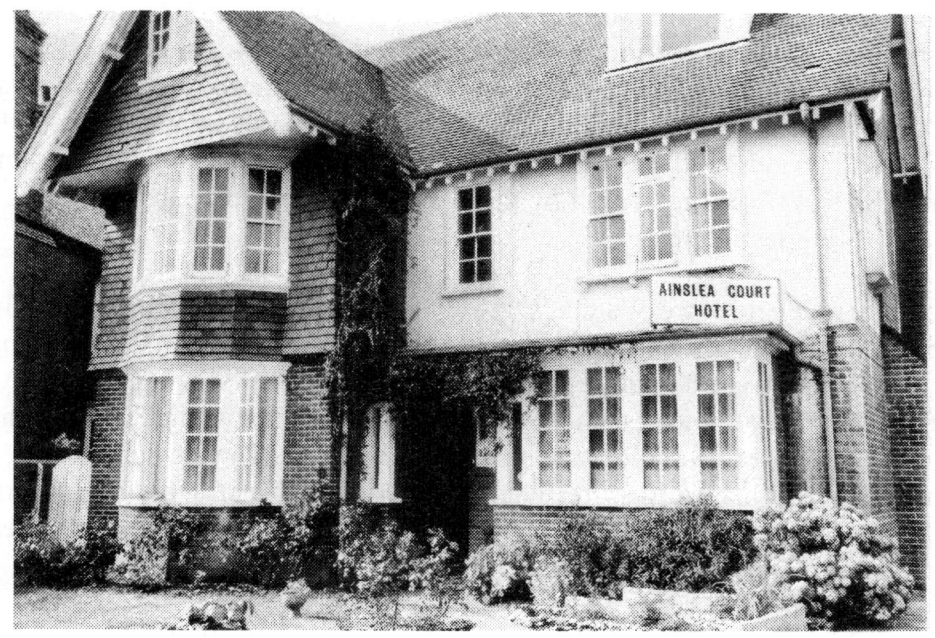

Ainsley Court

The holiday home continued in use for many years and the residents obviously enjoyed their visits. However, there are interesting hospital records that raise questions of how things functioned in practice. In 1983 there is an instruction to buy suitcases for residents going to Walton Hall and also a statement that the house lacks wardrobes and lockers!! This probably relates to the introduction at this time of personalised clothing. Prior to this date the Home would undoubtedly have retained a store of clothing, used by any person resident there at the time.

From the late 1950's until the 1980's Walton Hall was able to provide a holiday for approximately 380 people per year in groups of 20-21 at a time, increased to 30 with the construction of the bungalow for the Officer in Charge. However, it was decided in the mid-eighties that the home was too inconvenient. A new holiday home was bought by the Health Authority in early 1986. On the south coast, Ainsley Court in Worthing had been a small hotel. Mr. Roy Steele was appointed as the Officer in Charge. Walton Hall was sold in 1987.

The War Years.

In many records of Earlswood the staff and residents are described as 'the family'. There was a sense of closeness with and responsibility for all those associated with the Institution. This continues well into the twentieth century. Many of the male staff of Earlswood left their posts to fight in the Great War. Those who remained at home did not forget them. The Surrey Mirror of the 29th of December 1916 included a report of the Christmas festivities at Earlswood. According to this article all ex-staff on active duty were sent plum puddings. There is a report that an ex-attendant and the son of another attendant, who were both prisoners of war, were sent weekly food parcels.

In 1939 the London Office and Earlswood Home at Walton were both closed for the duration of the war and the buildings were requisition by the 'H. M. Principal Secretary of State for the War Department'. The office transferred to the Asylum and holidays ceased. Many other changes occurred at Earlswood. Blackouts were provided for all windows. A new six inch water main was laid to supply water for fire fighting should the need arise. In 1940 the fire station was reconstructed. Earlswood had its own air raid siren. There were no shelters built at Earlswood. However, internal blast walls were constructed, windows were bricked in or shutters were fitted and the basement corridor was sand bagged to provide a refuge for all during air raids. The following year fireproof screens and doors were placed on all stairways. Everyone at Earlswood was provided with a gas mask and in 1941 two decontamination units were purchased for managing victims of gas attacks. In 1942 the farmhouse on the Asylum farm in Lonesome Lane, Salfords was requisition by the War Department. The Institution was compensated at the rate of £130 per annum.

Male staff acted as volunteer air raid 'Fire Watchers', twelve per night in two-hour patrols. In 1940 there were nineteen attendants on active service, this had risen to 25 by the following year. In the first two years of the war 283 parcels had been sent to ex-staff serving abroad. As part of the effort to maintain moral amongst those in the armed forces awaiting action, the football pitch was made available on several occasions to military teams. The Asylum acquired 200 acres of extra land. Oak and ash trees were felled to provide timber for the war effort. Despite everything else there was still a waiting list for places at Earlswood. Long disused dormitories at the top of the main building were cleaned down and re-occupied

There were no war casualties at Earlswood. However, the building itself did not escape unscathed and the repairs to roofs, windows and doors cost in excess of £1,000. With the end of the war in 1945 the blast walls were removed and the blackout was taken down. The London Offices were released by the War Office and were let for three and a half years. The Earlswood Home at Walton was de-requisitioned.

There is evidence that, despite the horrors of the war itself, relatives of those at Earlswood did not forget their obligations to those at home. The Asylum Secretary received the following letter in 1944.

4th March 1944

'Dear Sir,

Mr. C. A. H. writes from Camp B.7.32 Yangehow, China under date 4th September 1943:- "Will you please communicate with the Earlswood

164

Institution that we are well and will remit funds when possible." Presumably correspondence is restricted by the Japanese and Mr. H. was unable to write to you direct.

Yours faithfully,

(Mrs) M. H. C.

Aunt of patient

The Secretary
The Royal Earlswood Institution
Redhill
Surrey

Post 1948.

Until 1948 the Asylum was an independent institution. However, the National Health Services Act transferred all hospitals to the Ministry of Health whilst leaving community care in the hands of local health authorities. On the 5th of July 1948, when the act became law, Earlswood became incorporated and was the parent unit in Group 43 in the South West Metropolitan Region under the administration of the Royal Earlswood Hospital Management Committee. Admission became free from the 1st of January 1948, replacing the system of election, part payment and full payment that had existed from the foundation of the Institution. Along with the hospital was transferred 175 acres of land.

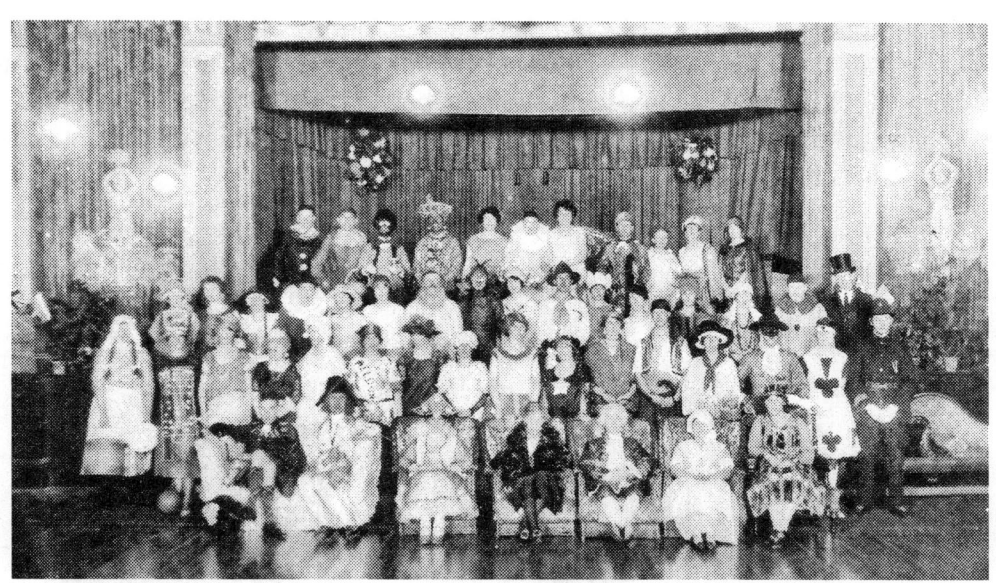

Concert

The other hospitals included in the group were Farmfield, previously administered by London County Council, and Forest Hospital at Horsham, previously a 'public assistance' institution managed by West Sussex County Council. The latter had fallen into disrepair during the war and held only 58 people with Learning Disability and 25 aged sick. Royal Earlswood undertook responsibility for those with Learning Disability in Sussex and shared responsibility with The Manor in Epsom for those in East Surrey. Farmfield was only for those from London initially. A Child Psychiatry Clinic was initiated in 1948.

With the reorganisation in 1974 Forest Hospital was transferred to the Cuckfield and Crawley District under the West Sussex Area Health Authority. Earlswood and Farmfield became members of the East Surrey Health District, part of Surrey Area Health Authority. The main hall at Royal Earlswood became a popular venue for many hospitals to hold functions. Farmfield closed in 1989 and Forest Hospital the following year. In 1997, three Assessment and Treatment Units were built at Farmfield following the closure of Earlswood.

Friends and Volunteers.

Earlswood from its earliest days relied on supporters and subscribers to provide for the needs of the residents. Over time the reliance on people to give annual subscriptions changed to a dependence on willing helpers prepared to donate time to aid residents or to raise funds. Many friends and family willingly directed their efforts to raising the residents' standard of living by providing extra comforts that could not be supplied initially from subscriptions and later from government funds.

The 'Friends' regularly raised money for projects at the Hospital to improve the lives of the residents. In 1974 the League of Friends provided £8,500 for the swimming pool. In 1975 they started a fund to restore the organ in the great hall, the restoration was completed in 1977. The League purchased wheelchairs for the Hospital and in 1978 provided a toy library that was open three days a week. In 1979 they contributed £5,000 for a mini-bus, a further £5,000 for a soft play area for adults and over £1,000 for play equipment.

As well as raising money the League of Friends organised outings for the residents and visited those who had no family nearby. They provided toys and games and also ensured that every resident had cards and gifts at Christmas and on their birthday. In October the Friends held an 'anniversary' party, attended in 1975 by the Mayor and Mayoress of Reigate, and there was also a party every Christmas.

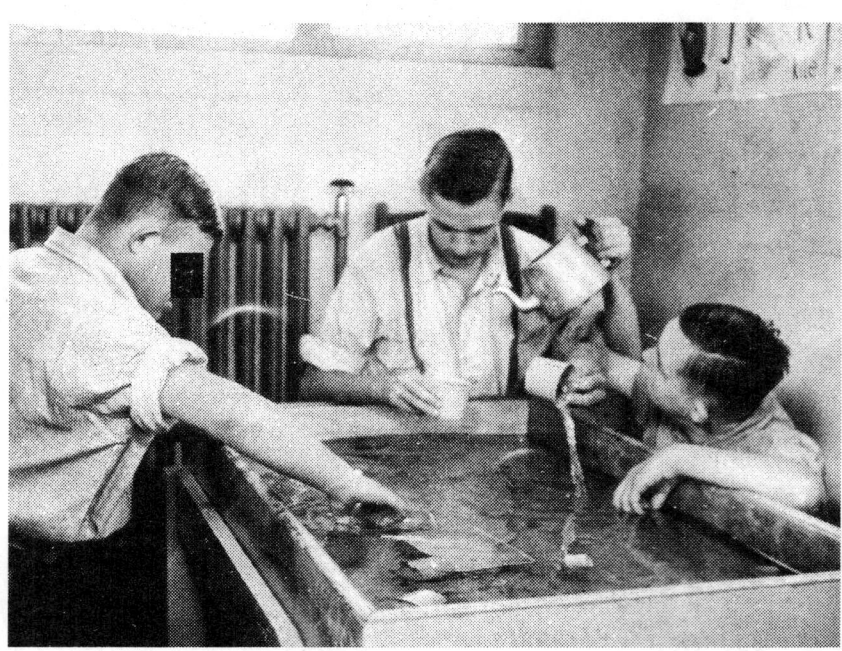

Sensory play

In addition to the 'Friends' there was also a place for volunteers to work within the Hospital, often one-to-one with the clients or organising leisure opportunities for them. In 1967 a consortium was formed to extend the scope of volunteer work. The members included the deputy chief male nurse, the assistant chief male nurse, the supervisor in occupational therapy and a senior psychologist. Later the matron joined the group. The consortium organised an annual sports day and bought the prizes.

There were, at the time, 130 volunteers. Twenty-one were individuals whilst the remainder belonged to schools, colleges, clubs, churches or other groups, 18 different organisations in all. Over 100 residents had regular contact with volunteers. Following several epidemics at the Hospital the number of volunteers declined alarmingly and a publicity campaign was launched. This proved so effective that by 1970 there were over 200 people regularly involved in volunteer work at Earlswood. A Volunteer Services Organiser, Mrs. B. M. Bashford, was appointed to co-ordinate the work of the volunteer 'army'.

Between 1967 and 1970 the list of voluntary activities was comprehensive, including:

Entertainments
Concerts, parties, plays, visits, dances, carols,
Sing-songs, country dancing, play groups during the holidays,
Help with fete day procession,
Making masks for drama group,
Taking patients out to tea,
Library,
Running hospital Womens' Institute,
Helping with sports,
Giving garden parties

Wards
Feeding patients,
Visiting patients,
Sweet Trolley
Exercising disabled children,
Pushing wheelchair patients out.

Education
Teaching typing,
Travel films and geography,
Art therapy,
Reading, arithmetic and money,
Music and movement,
Writing letters home,
Speech training,
Language development.

Physical Exercise
Swimming,
Athletics.

Technical Unit
General help and teaching,
Social training: traffic drill, shopping,
Hairdressing,
Beauty care,
Gardening.

Junior School
Giving extra attention to under-privileged children.

Non-patient Activities.
Cleaning,

Typing and filing,
Cataloguing,
Illuminated notices,
Repairing museum exhibits,
Making large toys and apparatus,
Advice on film editing,
Making costumes for drama group.

Miscellaneous.
Transport,
'Adopting' patients for birthday and Christmas presents.

In 1980 the League of Friends commissioned a film to be made about life at Earlswood. With a commentary by Brian Rix, the film was shown for the first time to staff on the 6th of December 1980.

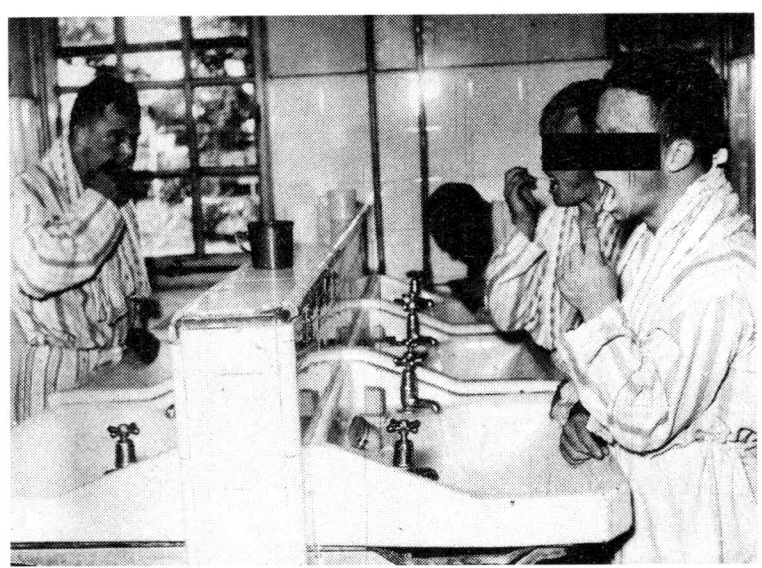

Daily life

A Name, a Charter and a Pledge.

'We plead for those who cannot plead for themselves'

The Charitable organisation, originally set up in 1847 as 'The Asylum for Idiots', was to have many names.

In 1862 Earlswood was incorporated by Royal Charter in the following terms.

'*Victoria,* by the Grace of God, of the United Kingdom of Great Britain and Ireland, Queen, Defender of the Faith.

To all to whom these presents shall come, greeting.

Whereas, in the year 1847, divers benevolent persons with the view of Improving the bodily and mental condition of Idiots and Imbeciles, formed Themselves into a Charitable Society under the name of "The Asylum for Idiots."

168

AND WHEREAS the better to enable the Society to carry their charitable Purposes into effect, they have erected and fitted up at Earlswood, near to Red Hill, in the county of Surrey, a building as an Asylum in which 400 Objects of the charity can be boarded, lodged and taken care of.

AND WHEREAS the benefits of the charity have already been extended to upwards of 800 idiots and imbeciles, and the number of them now in the Asylum at Earlswood is about 330, of whom about 160 are maintained there at the expense of the Society, about 100 are maintained there partly at the expense of the Society, and partly at the expense of their friends, and the others are maintained there at the expense of their friends.

AND WHEREAS besides their land and buildings at Earlswood the Society are entitled to the following trust estate, which came to them in the way of donation, that is to say, £500 South Eastern Railway Consolidated Stock; three £25 Shares in the Brighton and Hove Association for Improving the Dwellings of the Industrious Classes; and two £25 Shares in the London Association for the same object.

AND WHEREAS the property of the Society is vested in the names of trustees for the Society, and the trustees are a changing body and are removable at the will of the Society.

AND WHEREAS in order to carry into effect the benevolent intentions of the Society, it is requisite that in some instances contracts by or on the part of the Society to maintain idiots and imbeciles for life should be entered into, and in other cases contracts with respect to the removal or burial of idiots and imbeciles should be entered into by their friends............

AND WHEREAS our trusty and well-beloved James Abbiss, one of the Aldermen of our City of London, the Treasurer, and one of the members of the Board of Management of the Society, on behalf of himself and the Presidents, Vice-Presidents, and Board of Management of the Society, hath by his petition humbly besought us to grant to the Members of the Society our Royal Charter of Incorporation, for the purpose of promoting, securing, and extending the benevolent purposes of the Society.

NOW THEREFORE KNOW YE that we being graciously pleased to grant to the petitioner his request, and to give all fitting encouragement to the Society of our especial grace, certain knowledge and mere motion by these presents, for us, our heirs and successors, do grant, constitute and declare and appoint our trusty and well beloved the Baron Lionel de Rothschild; our trusty and well beloved the Reverend William Weldon Champneys, Clerk, M.A., and all such other person as now are and or hereafter shall become members of the Society, shall be and be called one body, politic and corporate in deed and in law by the name and style of "The Asylum for Idiots," and them by the name and style of "The Asylum for Idiots." ....

In Witness whereof we have caused these Our Letters to be made patent Witness ourself at our own Palace at Westminster this 25th day of November in the 26th year of our reign
    By Her Majesty's Command

'Mothers! Who know the heart's deep thrill
Of grateful, warm delight,
When little eyes have met thine own,
Intelligent and bright;
O feel for those poor human waifs
Cast on life's stormy tide,
And help the hands which thus have sought

This shelter to provide.

This Home, for which, in earnest voice,
'Tis Charity that pleads,
Son! Daughters! From your happier spheres,
And Heaven will send you recompense
From whence, nor slight, nor scorn
Nor aught but gentlest pitying love,
Beholds the IDIOT-BORN.

In 1902 it was noted that Earlswood was still the only national Asylum for the Learning Disabled. The continuing use of the term 'Idiot' was now considered to be unacceptable due to the derogatory sense of the term prevailing. The name was changed from the 'Earlswood Asylum' to the 'National Training Home for the Feeble-minded'.

In 1914 King George the Fifth granted Earlswood the right to use 'Royal' in its title and 'The Earlswood Asylum' changed its name to 'The Royal Earlswood Institution for Mental Defectives'.

In 1948, with the transfer of the Asylum to the National Health Service, the title of Royal Earlswood changed from 'Institution' to 'Hospital'.

The old Asylum motto is still true with a small modification,

We care for those who cannot care for themselves'

The Closure.

As early as 1929 there were calls for 'care in the community'. These gained impetus in the 1950s and 60s. By the 1970's there was an expansion in the development of community homes designed to receive residents of Earlswood felt to be capable of greater independence within the community. There was a range of abilities within Earlswood. For example 50-75 clients were recorded as capable of handling money, 250-300 could be cope with small amounts of money, whilst 200-250 were incapable of handling even the smallest amount of cash. As a halfway measure, clients moved into small units within the Earlswood site, such as the East Lodge in Princes Road.

From the units on site people moved to designated houses in the community supported by experienced staff, often with a long history of working at the Hospital. In this way there was a continuity of care but also a risk of institutionalisation outside of the Institution. One such staffed hostel was Redstone House that catered for 10 residents. The first four moved into the home on Monday the 15th of May 1978. The remaining six transferred a week later. Two homes opened in Greenways and Pollards Oak Rd, Hurst Green. These were smaller houses accommodating three and four persons respectively. Further group homes opened in Hardy Close, North Holmwood and Timperley Gardens, Redhill for three residents each. On the 14th of September 1979 it was announced that, due to health funding cuts, two wards at Earlswood were to close.

Indications of a change in attitude to large Institutions can be seen in 1984. In May of that year the size of many of the Homes at Earlswood was reduced, in some cases very significantly.

170

Dutch Villa was reduced by eight beds, from 30 to 22, Albert Home reduced by seven beds, from 38 to 31. Farm Villa reduced by six beds, Alice Unit and Alexandra reduced by four, Charles and Anne Homes by three. Phillip, Mark and Elizabeth each lost two beds, Marina, Henry, Margaret, Andrew Reed and Brook House reduced by one each.

Respite care had initially been provided within the Institution but this was now seen as less acceptable and Daffodil House was opened on the 22nd of September 1989 to provide short-term care in place of Louise Ward. Shortly before this, on the 14th of July 1989, ten rooms had been made available at 18-20 Princes Road, for occupation by clients or staff.

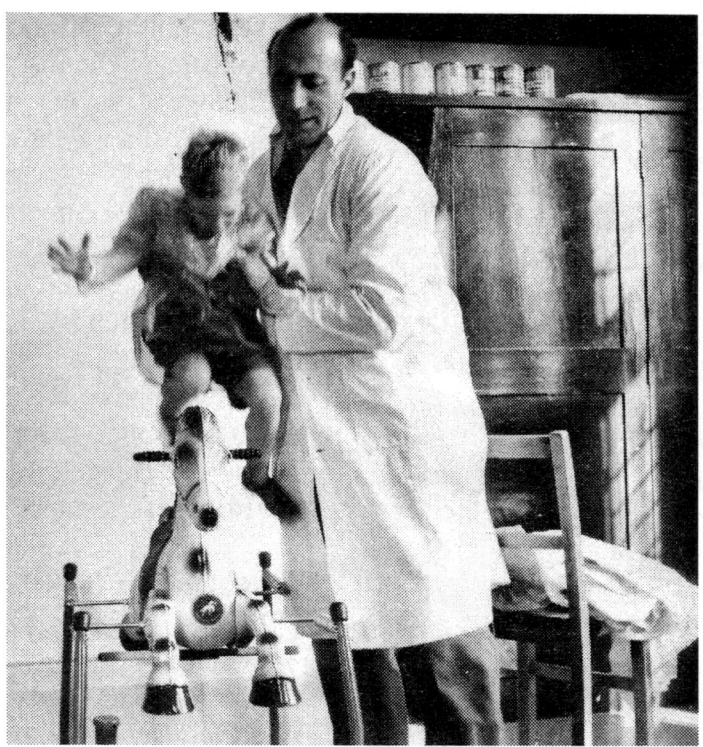

Having fun!

The transfer of clients into the community continued throughout the nineties with the more able being transferred first. By 1994 there were about 290 residents still remaining in the Hospital. At this time the final three-year closure program began. Three options were available for community provision. Approximately 50 clients were identified to move into Assessments and Treatment Units that were to be designated as inpatient provision. One hundred clients would move into homes owned by housing associations and staffed by Surrey Oaklands NHS Trust or other care agencies. The remainder would be accommodated in private care homes, some pre-existing and others specially set up. Many of those in Earlswood were not from Surrey, 45% originated from out of county. In some cases the home authority or the family requested that resettlement took place in the home county. Homes were found in Devon, Northamptonshire, Yorkshire, Buckinghamshire, in all corners of the British Isles.

The final closure of Earlswood occurred on the 31st of March 1997. In the final month 120 clients were moved into their new homes in the community.

Index